The metaphor of mental illness

International Perspectives in Philosophy and Psychiatry

Series editors

Bill (K. W. M.) Fulford
Katherine Morris
John Z Sadler
Giovanni Stanghellini

Volumes in the series:

Mind, Meaning, and Mental Disorder
Bolton and Hill

Nature and Narrative: An Introduction to the New Philosophy of Psychiatry
Fulford, Morris, Sadler, and Stanghellini

Dementia: Mind, Meaning, and the Person
Hughes, Louw, and Sabat (ed.)

The Philosophy of Psychiatry: A Companion
Radden

Values and Psychiatric Diagnosis
Sadler

Disembodied Spirits and Deanimated Bodies: The Psychopathology of Common Sense
Stanghellini

Forthcoming volumes in the series:

Postpsychiatry
Bracken and Thomas

The Philosophical Understanding of Schizophrenia
Chung, Fulford, and Graham (ed.)

The Oxford Textbook of Philosophy and Psychiatry
Fulford, Thornton, and Graham

The metaphor of mental illness

Neil Pickering
Lecturer,
Bioethics Centre,
University of Otago,
Dunedin,
New Zealand

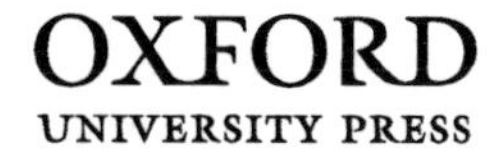

OXFORD
UNIVERSITY PRESS

Great Clarendon Street, Oxford OX2 6DP

Oxford University Press is a department of the University of Oxford.
It furthers the University's objective of excellence in research, scholarship,
and education by publishing worldwide in

Oxford New York

Auckland Cape Town Dar es Salaam Hong Kong Karachi
Kuala Lumpur Madrid Melbourne Mexico City Nairobi
New Delhi Shanghai Taipei Toronto

With offices in

Argentina Austria Brazil Chile Czech Republic France Greece
Guatemala Hungary Italy Japan Poland Portugal Singapore
South Korea Switzerland Thailand Turkey Ukraine Vietnam

Oxford is a registered trade mark of Oxford University Press
in the UK and in certain other countries

Published in the United States
by Oxford University Press Inc., New York

First published 2006

British Library Cataloguing in Publication Data

Data available

Library of Congress Cataloging in Publication Data

Data available

Typeset by Newgen Imaging Systems (P) Ltd., Chennai, India
Printed in Great Britain
on acid-free paper by
Biddles Ltd., King's Lynn

ISBN 0–19–853087–0 (Hbk.) 978–0–19–853087–9 (Hbk.)
ISBN 0–19–853088–9 (Pbk.) 978–0–19–853088–6 (Pbk.)

10 9 8 7 6 5 4 3 2 1

To my parents

Acknowledgements

This book has taken shape over the period of 15 years or so, and in that time many people have had a significant influence on my ideas and have offered intellectual support, and challenge. Professor Donald Evans has been a constant source of all these, and has done everything he can to provide me with the opportunity to study, teach, and research these topics, first in Swansea, and later in New Zealand. Professor Martyn Evans and Dr David Greaves were supervisors of my PhD, upon which much of this book is based: without them there would have been no PhD and hence no book. Other members of the staff and students of the Centre for the Study of Philosophy and Health Care at the University of Wales, Swansea, and of the Department of Philosophy there, provided a stimulating intellectual atmosphere. Latterly, I've benefited in a similar way in the University of Otago, in the Bioethics Centre and the Department of Psychological Medicine in particular. Professor K.W.M. (Bill) Fulford has also always been a tremendous source of support and encouragement, and so too, latterly, has Professor Grant Gillett. A number of anonymous referees made very useful suggestions about how I might develop the original proposal for this book.

Nothing like this gets done without personal support and I've been blessed with this from Don and Anne Evans, Martyn and Jan Evans, David and Pat Greaves, Lynley Anderson, Claire Gallop, Chikako Maruyama, and more recently Fiona Pickering and Donald and Stella Cullington. The book is dedicated, with all my love and gratitude, to my parents.

I have benefited from a number of sources of financial or other support: The Religious Society of Friends (Quakers) Social Responsibility and Education section gave me a grant to help me study in Swansea and I also received financial support from the Centre for the Study of Philosophy and Health Care. The University of Otago gave me a period of study leave during which much work was done to prepare the manuscript.

Two chapters in this book have been substantially published previously. Chapter 5 appeared as Metaphors and Models in Medicine in Theoretical Medicine and Bioethics (1999, volume 20, pp.361–375); I would like to thank the publishers and editors of TMB for permission to use this material. The article and hence this chapter benefited immensely from the comments of the anonymous referees of TMB, particularly one of them. Chapter 2 appeared as The Likeness Argument and the Reality of Mental Illness in Philosophy, Psychiatry and Psychology (2003, volume 10, Number 3, pp.243–254); I would like the thank the publishers and editors of PPP for permission to use this material.

Given the amount of help I've received, there really shouldn't be any errors or mistakes in the book: however, I've absolutely no doubt that I've managed to perpetrate numbers of these, and for them I take sole responsibility.

NP
October, 2005

Contents

1 Introduction: the existence of mental illness

1.1 The sceptical challenge

'My aim in this essay is to raise the question "Is there such a thing as mental illness?" and to argue that there is not' (Szasz, 1982, p. 19). Questions like this one, which Thomas Szasz posed first in 1960, are the starting point for this book. According to Szasz mental illness is a myth (as in the title of the article the above quote is taken from) or a metaphor. According to Mary Boyle (1990), schizophrenia is a 'scientific delusion'. According to Breggin (1998) there's no such illness as ADHD.

The aim of this book is to explore one way in which it is possible to answer Szasz's radical question with a yes. This way of answering yes is to say that mental illness, or specific diagnoses, exist in so far as we create or invent them. This way of answering takes seriously the underlying reasons for the scepticism of some who ask these radical questions and answer them with a no. Indeed, in putting forward this way of answering yes I shall accept a good deal of what the sceptics say. Indeed, I imagine that some reading this book will sense that I accept a good deal too much of the sceptics' arguments. Often I shall suggest, for example, that we can accept pretty much all of what a sceptic claims, but still reach a non-sceptical conclusion.

What underlies the position explored here is a sense that the reasons both sceptics and non-sceptics typically give for their answers to the radical questions are faulty. There's something wrong about the way the debate has in large part been set up, something misleading about the choices we are commonly offered. We need to rethink the debate.

1.2 Why is the debate important?

As concepts or ideas, such things as mental illness, schizophrenia, and ADHD are entrenched in the language, institutions, and constitutions of many countries. Take English-speaking countries: in everyday English we find both lay terms such as 'nervous breakdown' that relate to mental illness as a whole, and terms related in various ways to specific psychiatric diagnoses such as 'schizo' and 'pscyho'. Stories that have got into the public eye have made paranoid schizophrenia, psychopathy, Munchausen's syndrome by proxy and post-traumatic stress disorder familiar terms. Anorexia and bulimia afflict or are said to afflict actresses (Calista Flockhart for example) and princesses (Princess Diana most famously). Factual accounts such as *Tell Me I'm Here* (Deveson, 1992) or Janet Frame's autobiography (Frame, 1990) in the case of schizophrenia, give lay readers an insight into the experience of people who are, or are labelled, or who care for those who are said to be mentally ill. So do literary works such as *Briefing For A Descent Into Hell* (Lessing, 1971) and *One Flew Over the Cuckoo's Nest* (Kesey, 1973). The latter was made into a film (Forman, 1975). Then there are the endless jokes about the schizophrenic in two minds (a popular misunderstanding of schizophrenia) or those who think they are ducks, dogs, and so on.

The often vast buildings sometimes of nineteenth century origin in which the mentally ill were housed and treated are also an element of the general consciousness and became treated with fear and ignorance. Elaine Murphy remembers a psychiatric hospital from her childhood: 'Mapperley—the very name was awesome to me. It meant the asylum, the "looney bin", the "nut house", a massive, gloomy red-brick institution where crazy, peculiar people lived secret, mysterious lives.' (Murphy, 1991, p. 1; for some similar reactions see Frame, 1990, p. 150).

Alongside these lay understandings are specialist, usually medical, understandings of mental illnesses, and all the associated institutions and roles that go with these. In addition to asylums such as Mapperley, there are psychiatric prisons, psychiatric wings attached to District General Hospitals, half-way houses, and other community institutions. There are units that specialize in disorders such as anorexia nervosa and ADHD. There is the entire panoply of psychiatry itself, from education and training institutions, to specialist journals, and the Royal College (in UK) and its equivalents elsewhere (the American Psychiatric Association for example). Working with psychiatrists are mental health specialists from other fields: psychiatric nurses, psychiatric social workers, educational psychologists. Working in the same field there are campaigning groups such as MIND, NSF (The National Schizophrenia Fellowship in the UK), and CHADD (Children and Adults with Attention Deficit Hyperactivity Disorder, a US group). Interventions said to be for the control, treatment, and cure of mental illness have been developed. These range from electroconvulsive therapy and surgical interventions such as lobotomy, to drugs. Chlorpromazine (Largactil) and other neuroleptics have been developed for use with schizophrenia and mania, and antidepressants for use with depression (Healy, 1990, p. 65). The brand names of some of these drugs have become household names: Prozac (used in depression) and Ritalin (used in ADHD) to name but a couple.

Beyond the common stock of language and the medical institutions, mental illness has a role in the legal and constitutional structure of many jurisdictions. The UK is a good example again. The concept is enshrined in the UK Mental

Health Act of 1983 (Jones, 1984), in the justice system, and in the fabric of political rights. Those who have a mental illness and are being treated for it are one group who may not sit on juries (Hoggett, 1996, p. 227). Within the common law, those of unsound mind and 'idiots' may neither vote in nor stand for an election (*ibid.*, p. 225). There is a statutory procedure for vacating the seat of an MP who has been detained compulsorily under the Mental Health Act 1983 for more than 6 months (*ibid.*, p. 227). At the same time as certain rights are taken away, so too are certain kinds of responsibility. Within the justice system, the McNaghten rules enshrine a legal notion that someone who is not in a state of mind to face trial or was not capable of telling the difference between right and wrong at the time of the alleged crime, should not be charged or should be found not-guilty. A psychiatrist is often called in to testify on the subject of state of mind. This formal benefit is reflected in the informal benefits of not bearing responsibility for one's acts or failings if a mental illness explains them. Many people, for example, welcome a diagnosis of ADHD because it tells them that they are not to blame. Elliott reports one adult ADHD sufferer as saying 'I had 38 years of thinking I was a bad person . . . Now I'm rewriting the tapes of who I thought I was to who I really am' (2003, p. 256; see also Diller, 1998, pp. 125–6). Moreover, illness is generally a gateway to entitlements of one sort or another. Mental illness is no exception. Children with ADHD may be eligible for special education services (Cohen, nd.; Fukuyama, 2002, p. 50). Diagnoses of post-traumatic stress disorder may be used to apply for benefits as a result of exposure to traumatizing events (Vietnam Veterans of America, 2004). On the other hand, to be diagnosed with a mental illness is also widely regarded as stigmatizing and ostracizing.

In short, the notion of mental illness, and many specific mental illness diagnoses are deeply entrenched in the day-to-day fabric of ordinary lives, and in the medical, legal, and constitutional arrangements of developed Western societies such as the UK.

So, the fact that there are those who deny altogether that mental illness exists is interesting and important, as is the fact that there are numerous writers who deny that particular diagnoses are legitimate. Just because mental illness is so entrenched and far reaching an idea, these denials are challenging. If it were right to deny the existence of mental illness altogether, for example, this would force a fundamental review of many of the arrangements of countries around the world, and many of their people's beliefs. It would be a revolutionary change. However, it would not be without precedent. Szasz reminds us that a set of similarly entrenched concepts, language uses, and social institutions once existed, which now seem to most based upon a fiction. He has in mind witchcraft (Szasz, 1973). Those who deny the very existence of mental illness, claim we should deny the legitimacy of the panoply of psychiatry and by implication all else that depends on the idea, just as society generally now denies witchcraft and all that relied upon it. Even if we restrict our selves to scepticism about specific diagnoses, some of these are well-established enough to have a similar sort of impact—schizophrenia for example. And to deny the legitimacy of even a relatively recent diagnosis such as ADHD would have an impact on the many people who, in one way and another, have organized aspects of their lives and beliefs around its supposed existence. It is such radical outright denials which I will focus on in what follows.

1.3 Radical questions and radical cures

We should distinguish such outright denial from radical approaches to mental illnesses to be found within or on the fringes of psychiatry and psychology (cf. Jenner *et al.*, 1993), from campaigns against the abuse of certain techniques within psychiatry, and from at least some versions of the antipsychiatry position. I shall not be concerned with these in this book.

To seek to radicalize a treatment approach is not necessarily to deny that the object of the treatment is still mental illness. Anthony Clare wrote the foreword to Jenner *et al.* and is able to endorse much of what the book says as a corrective to narrowly biological views of schizophrenia. However, he does not go so far as to give up the view that 'schizophrenia or the schizophrenias are probably best categorised as disease' (Clare, 1993, p. 7). Diller, who is a thoughtful critique of ADHD, argues that the diagnosis is often a substitute for something that would be more appropriate, a change of parenting style, or of expectations of a child, for example (1998, e.g. pp. 75ff). However, he does not go so far as to deny the illness status of a central core of children said to have ADHD.

But sceptics such as Szasz do not think that psychiatrists have focused in an untoward manner on biological accounts of mental illness. For the radical sceptic, mental illness being non-existent, there is nothing for psychiatrists to have focused too narrowly on. To campaign against the abuses of the system is not necessarily to question its legitimacy within certain moral limits. Szasz complains, he tells us, of the abuse that *is* psychiatry (Szasz, 1973, pp. 24–5). And for someone like Breggin a similar analysis can be made in the case of a specific diagnosis, namely, ADHD. For him ADHD is simply an excuse for drugging children into conformity with society's expectations and to make life easy for teachers and parents and various educational and other institutions.

Historically, Szasz is sometimes associated with the antipsychiatry movement;[1] Pilgrim (1992) lists him among others. Pilgrim also lists Peter Sedgwick, but Sedgwick is critical of Szasz, and seeks to distance himself from him. Szasz, Sedgwick (1982) says, employs a 'mechanical and inaccurate' medical model. The crux of Sedgwick's position is stated here:

> Quite correctly, the anti-psychiatrists have pointed out that psychopathological categories refer to value judgements and that mental illness is deviancy.

> On the other hand, the anti-psychiatric critics themselves are wrong when they imagine physical medicine to be essentially different in its logic from psychiatry. A diagnosis of diabetes, or paresis, includes the recognition of norms or values. Anti-psychiatry can only operate by positing a mechanical and inaccurate model of physical illness and its medical diagnosis. It follows, therefore, from the above train of argument that mental illnesses can be conceptualised within the disease framework just as easily as physical maladies such as lumbago or TB. Sedgwick (1982, p. 56)

Here Sedgwick argues that the difference between psychiatry and physical medicine upon which he believes Szasz relies is a chimera. Sedgwick agrees with Szasz that the logic of mental illness entails a social value judgement. However, Sedgwick does not see this as a reason to object to the category of mental illness. Rather, in this respect mental illness is logically the same as physical illness. Nor is it a reason to object to psychiatry, except and in so far as psychiatry insists on a certain technologized and mechanical view of mental illness. For as much and the same could be said of physical illness. Sedgwick, then, aims at reform of psychiatry through clarification of concepts such as mental illness. This cannot be Szasz's programme, as Sedgwick recognizes. From Szasz's point of view, one cannot reform but only abolish what is itself an abuse, nor clarify one's understanding of what is non-existent (though one can clarify the fact that it is non-existent).

Szasz, then, is quite different from others identified as antipsychiatrists. Sedgwick rejects a technologized mechanical view of mental illness, but thinks it can be 'conceptualised within the disease framework' as easily as TB; Szasz rejects the idea that mental illness, in so far as it is a medical category, has any reality. Szasz's opposition to psychiatry has often meant he is thought of as one of the antipsychiatry group. He is only in the sense that antipsychiatry objects to traditional medicalized psychiatry. Szasz is a conceptual radical: his opposition to psychiatry is a root and branch opposition. The very foundation of psychiatry, the existence of its object of study and of treatment and cure, is what Szasz denies. This is the kind of radicalism I am interested in and this book represents an attempt to reconsider what it means and how to counter it.

When it comes to the level of specific diagnoses, similar sorts of contrast can be drawn. ADHD is a good example. Writers who are critical of the degree of medicalization of, say, ADHD include Carl Elliott (2003), Francis Fukuyama (2002), Peter Conrad (1976),[2] Laurence Diller (who we have already mentioned), and many others. These writers are concerned among other things with the amount of drugs being given to young people in the name of the diagnosis. They all observe cases where children who are only very questionably suffering from ADHD are given drugs rather than time being taken to look at them and the context of their lives more carefully and fully. However, none of these writers is tempted to go quite so far as to say that ADHD is altogether a fiction. They recognize abuses, but someone like

Breggin takes the much more radical line that the whole idea of ADHD is abusive. Likewise, Mary Boyle is a radical when it comes to the existence of schizophrenia. While Jenner *et al.*. seek to redefine approaches to schizophrenia, she says it is a fiction invented by psychiatrists such as Bleuler and Kraepelin. For her, there is nothing to redefine our approaches to.

1.4 Response to the radical questions

I am far from being the first person to try to respond to radical questions such as those posed by Szasz, Breggin, or Boyle. Many of those who have thought about the nature of mental illness over the past 30 years or so have seen it as important to take Szasz particularly into account. So this book seeks to stand in a tradition that runs from Flew, through Boorse, Sedgwick, Fulford, Reznek, Wakefield, and many others. All of these writers take Szasz's challenge seriously, and have sought to answer his radical question (and all of them have answered yes to it).

In joining this list, I want to ask what sort of questions these radical questions are: what sort of question is *does mental illness exist*; what sort of questions are *does schizophrenia* and *does ADHD exist*. My approach will be somewhat in the spirit of a remark made by Wittgenstein: 'show me *how* you are searching and I will tell you *what* you are looking for' (1975, p. 67). My question about the radical questions is: what *sort* of answer do these questions ask for? How we may go about seeking to answer Szasz's question or other radical questions about specific diagnoses tells us what sort of question they have been taken to be.

My argument in the first part of this book will be that one very large tradition of attempts to answer these radical questions is based upon particular, but mistaken, assumptions about the nature of the question. This tradition relies on what I shall call the likeness argument. This argument is, in brief and general terms, that we can prove or disprove the existence of mental illness or the validity of some particular diagnostic category such as schizophrenia or ADHD by showing or discovering whether such human conditions are or are not illnesses. We do this, the likeness argument says, by showing that schizophrenia or ADHD are or are not sufficiently similar to other illnesses to be illnesses themselves. The assumption about the question upon which the likeness argument is based is that it is answerable by evidence as to the nature of the conditions in question which is available to observation. It assumes that if we observe or investigate conditions such as schizophrenia, alcoholism, ADHD, or bipolar affective disorder for the features of illness, then this will decide for us whether or not these are illnesses. If upon investigation it turns out that conditions such as schizophrenia do have the features of illness, it will be possible to say that mental illness exists; if ADHD turns out to have the features of illness, it will be possible to say that it is an illness.

The significance of this means of trying to answer radical questions, at least for the purposes of this book, is that it removes—or appears to remove—from the answer the role of what we might call human agency. This is the point of making the answer to the question a matter of discovery and observation of how things are. On closer inspection, however, it turns out that the question cannot after all be answered in this way. My argument will be that the likeness argument is circular and that when we realize this we see that, and indeed where human agency must come in. The features of conditions, such as schizophrenia, alcoholism, or ADHD, which the likeness argument relies upon to decide what kind of thing they are change depending upon one's conceptualization of these conditions. For example, it might be thought that if the behaviours in alcoholism are causally related to brain abnormalities this will show that alcoholism is an illness and not a failure of character. Or it might be supposed that if the thought processes of schizophrenics arise from dysfunctions of the brain or mind rather than simply representing strange ideas and beliefs, then this suggests that schizophrenia is an illness. If alcoholism and schizophrenia are like this it seems to prove or strongly support the case that they are illnesses. We expect illnesses to be describable in causal and functional terms. However, I shall argue that the causal and dysfunctional features of schizophrenia and alcoholism are created in the light of the kind of thing they are thought to be. If one thinks they are illnesses, they will appear to have features such as causal brain abnormalities; but if one does not think they are illnesses these features will be absent. It is the argument of this book that this is the role that human agency plays in mental illness: it is responsible for categorizing conditions as illnesses, and thereby making the features of illness such as causality or dysfunction appear.

The likeness argument makes the assumption that the idea that there are mental illnesses—or that conditions such as schizophrenia are examples of mental illness—makes sense. It is only because of this assumption that it makes sense to think it is possible to discover mental illnesses, or find out whether something is or is not a mental illness. However, we can raise a question about whether the notion of mental illness is intelligible. The sceptic says no—the very idea of mental illness ought to be abandoned. Nothing can be a mental illness, the sceptic argues, because mental illness is an incoherent idea. It involves putting together two other ideas that do not fit with one another. Nothing could be both 'mental' and 'ill'. I propose to accept something of this claim but without reaching the conclusion that it seems most naturally to lead to. (As I mentioned earlier, the book tends to accept a good deal of what the sceptic argues without necessarily being sceptical itself.) I accept that the combination of 'mental' and 'ill' is indeed conceptually challenging. The argument of this book is indeed that mental illness is a combination of ideas that do not fit. It is a human categorization of phenomena that seem best to be described in evaluative (social, political, moral) terms into a different category where other descriptive terms (cause, dysfunction) are to be found. In short, it is a metaphor.

Interestingly, this is just what sceptic Thomas Szasz says about mental illness. However, in his mind, to call mental illness a metaphor is tantamount to being a sceptic. Sceptics think that metaphor is a deceptive thing, and that it involves simply playing with words. I suggest that it does not necessarily involve any form of deception. It involves categorization, and this categorization is imaginative—it is not based upon existing uses of words or applications of categories. For this reason metaphors may sound odd or wrong (Aristotle says they involve wrong naming). However, it is in this apparent wrongness that it can be seen that the imagination is working to create something new. When we look at uses of metaphor in medical science outside psychiatry—at Pasteur's use of metaphor in the case of vaccination, for example (in Chapter 5)—we see how it creates new categories and new possibilities of description. On a wider scale, that of the idea that the human body is a machine, something similar appears. To say that the body is a machine is a metaphor (in my view): it is a categorization that is odd. However, on the basis of this categorization, specific machine analogies for various parts and actions of the body—such as vocalizing—are made possible.

This is the nature of the human agency, which I believe the likeness argument tries and fails to keep out of the picture. Just as Pasteur made what we now call vaccination, and the enlightenment thinkers made the body a machine, so humans make mental illness and make conditions such as ADHD and schizophrenia into illnesses. Mental illness is the product of human thinking. It is a historical fact about human thinking that it has developed this category and produced mental illnesses, ADHD, schizophrenia, and so on.

In the third part of the book we turn to mental illness and to the implications of the view being putting forward. In Chapters 6 and 7 are examples of what this broad claim might mean in two specific contexts. The first is the development of the modern idea of mental illness, around the first half of the nineteenth century. The second is the development of the idea of ADHD. To try to understand what my claims mean, in considering these two examples, I seek to contrast my view with different possible forms of the sceptical view. For example, the development of the idea of mental illness after 1800 or so can be analysed in terms offered us by the strong programme in the sociology of knowledge; and the development of the idea of ADHD can be analysed from the perspective of social constructionism. Both these views can be developed sceptically, and both are quite close to the view of this book.

What both views do is to propose a history that demonstrates—or claims to demonstrate—the origins of the categorization in human processes. Both suggest that what is pictured by psychiatrists as a natural or perhaps objective feature of the world is actually a creation of psychiatry or, more broadly, the society in which psychiatry thrives or at least has developed. In each case a broad socio-economic or political background is held to be reflected in and to be responsible for the existence of the categorization. These views lend themselves to scepticism: By the standards normally set by science, the fact that

these are human products appears to render mental illness or whatever particular diagnoses are involved, highly suspicious. They do not reflect the world of nature, as you would expect diseases to do—they are not its products: rather they seem to be the products of humans.

My response—slightly differently worked out in the two cases—is that scepticism is not the logical outcome of such views. Such views are right to say that the category of mental illness and specific mental illness diagnoses are human products. And they are right to say that it is only in the light of the categorization of conditions as illnesses that features such as genetic causality and so on appear. However, the sceptical conclusion does not follow because the relations between these ideas, and these ideas themselves, are not of a social nature. Rather, they are of a medical scientific character. Medical science has developed a set of ideas and theorizations. It seeks to understand things such as so-called mental illness and ADHD in specific medical ways. I argue that neither the strong programme in the sociology of knowledge, nor the social constructionist account, manages to show that mental illness and ADHD are constructed in any way other than medically. The sceptical case relies, I think, on showing that these ideas are actually constructed out of political, moral, or economic beliefs and values. But this it does not do. Because they are constructed out of what are medical features of the world it is possible to carry these ideas into the brain, and other such areas of the world.

So, I shall argue, the answer to Thomas Szasz's radical question *does mental illness exist* can be yes. It exists in virtue of the fact that it is a work of human imagination. This imagination is focused on features of the world that appear within the scientific approach to biology and psychology. But that is not tantamount to saying mental illness or illnesses do not exist after all. Rather, that is how they exist.

Endnotes

1 The label antipsychiatry initially refers to the ideas and practice of R.D. Laing and his followers. For example, David Cooper acknowledges a deep debt to Laing in his book *Psychiatry and Anti-Psychiatry* (Cooper, 1970; first published in 1967). A text first published in 1971 is called *Laing and Anti-Psychiatry* (Boyers and Orrill, 1972). The association of Szasz (and Foucault) with antipsychiatry is noted by Goldstein in the entry on 'Psychiatry' in Bynum and Porter (1993, p. 1368). Ian Hacking pointed out to me that a number of texts, including important early ones by Laing and Szasz, came out around the same time, but were produced independently. Laing's *The Divided Self* (Laing, 1964) was first published in 1960; Szasz's article 'The Myth of Mental Illness' (Szasz, 1982) was published in 1960, and his book of the same name first appeared in 1961 (Szasz, 1974a); Foucault's *Madness and Civilisation* was first published in English in 1965, but *Histoire de la Folie* was published in 1961 in French; and Goffman's *Asylums* first appeared in 1961. Pilgrim (1992) records two generations of historians critical of psychiatry. In addition to Szasz and Foucault, he

includes Scull (1979) in the first. The second generation includes Foucault's followers (Castel *et al.*, 1979; Castel, 1983; Miller and Rose, 1986) and Baruch and Treacher (1978), Ingleby (1981, 1983), Sedgwick (1982), and Ramon (1985). For an account of the British antipsychiatry movement and further sources see Crossley (1998).

2 Conrad's book of 1976 is a sociological investigation of hyperactivity, plausibly an earlier name (one of several, perhaps) for what is now labelled ADHD. Conrad has continued to write in this field, for example in Conrad and Potter (2000).

Part 1

Answering radical questions

[S]how me how you are searching and I will tell you what you are looking for

(Wittgenstein, 1975, p. 67)

2 The likeness argument

2.1 Introduction

In the previous chapter some radical questions were identified: *Does mental illness exist? Is schizophrenia an illness?* This book explores an answer—and a justification for that answer—to these questions. The answer to be explored will be yes: but its justification will be close—perilously close some might say—to the kind of justification used by those who answer no. It is, in short, that mental illness exists—and that specific illnesses such as schizophrenia, alcoholism, and ADHD exist—as a result of human agency: we make or produce them. This may seem a quite inappropriate basis of existence for things that are conceived of in illness or disease terms: it looks more like a basis for denying them existence. However, I aim to show that we are forced into taking this foundation for mental illness up when we see that—and more especially how—the existing attempts to answer the radical questions must fail to do so.

The majority of attempts to answer these radical questions have taken the same route. This route is an attempt to prove (or disprove) the existence of mental illness, by showing that certain conditions—say schizophrenia—are illnesses (or are not illnesses, as the case may be) because they are sufficiently (or insufficiently) like some other condition everyone agrees is an illness—say pneumonia or cancer. This route concentrates on the features of so-called mental illnesses (e.g. schizophrenia) and compares them with those of physical illnesses. Provided these features are similar, the argument holds, the mental disturbances or conditions will also rank as illnesses. This of course directly resolves questions such as *Is schizophrenia an illness* and by extension starts to answer the wider question about mental illness as a whole.

I will refer to this route to answering the radical questions as the likeness argument. This chapter asks: can the likeness argument hope to achieve what it seems intended to achieve by those who employ it, namely to answer the radical questions one way or the other? This chapter raises a doubt about whether it can hope to do so. The source of this doubt is fundamental to the argument of the book. The likeness argument seeks to answer the radical questions by reference to the features of putative mental illnesses, such as schizophrenia. It restricts the role of humans to investigating what the features of conditions such as schizophrenia and ADHD are. However, this chapter will suggest that humans play a much more active role than that.

Some issues in setting out

The doubt about the ability of the likeness argument to settle the disputes it sets out to settle is such that it applies equally to all those using the likeness argument. The likeness argument is overwhelmingly often used to answer the radical questions I raised previously in the affirmative. 'Yes', those who use the likeness argument most often argue, 'mental illness does exist', or 'yes, that particular behavioural pattern or condition is an illness' (e.g. it is rightly designated ADHD, alcoholism, schizophrenia). However, it can equally well be used to argue the opposite. The problem with the likeness argument which will be raised lies with the form of the argument and not its conclusion. Hence, the doubts about the likeness argument expressed in this chapter will not favour a sceptic such as Szasz, who is well known for his answer to his own radical question, namely that mental illness has no reality and is a socially convenient medical myth. Nor will it help sceptics about specific disorders, such as Breggin in the case of ADHD. If Breggin or Szasz use a likeness argument to argue their cases, it must fail them just as it fails the numerous others who use it to argue for the opposite conclusions, and for exactly similar reasons.

Nor does this chapter seek to take sides on the many other issues that divide those who use the likeness argument. This is not to deny the importance of these issues. For example, Boorse (1977, 1982) differs in several quite marked ways from Fulford (1989). Significantly, they understand their target concepts quite differently: Boorse aims to determine whether or not there is such a thing as mental *disease*, whereas Fulford aims for the concept *illness*. Theirs are not merely terminological disputes, as Boorse means something quite different by disease than Fulford means by illness (or Wakefield (1992a,b) by disorder, or Culver and Gert (1982) by malady, or Brody (1985) by sickness).

None the less, important though these issues are they are not relevant to the argument of this chapter. Its aim is to throw doubt on the ability of the likeness argument to work, whatever concept is worked with. This chapter suggests that the problem lies in the form of the argument, not in its specific content. For ease the term illness will be used most often in the remainder of this chapter and indeed throughout the book; however, no particular content is assigned to it. When the time comes to consider the arguments of a specific writer, whatever term she or he uses will be employed.

2.2 The likeness argument

Two forms of the likeness argument

The likeness argument says that so-called mental illnesses will rightly be classified or categorized as illnesses to the extent that these conditions have the features of illnesses; and to the extent they lack these features, classifying them as illnesses will be a mistake. As I said earlier, it directly answers radical questions about specific claimed diagnoses (questions such as is schizophrenia an illness? or is ADHD an illness?). And it uses answers to these questions to answer the wider radical question does mental illness exist?

In the literature there are a number of variations of the likeness argument, but these turn out to be compatible with one another. The two main versions can be labelled the paradigm and the generic approaches. The starting point for the paradigm form of the argument is best summed up by Boorse, who says that 'a legitimate notion of mental health must be a faithful analogue of the established physical conception' (1977, p. 543; cf. also Boorse, 1982). Health, for Boorse, is simply the absence of disease. Boorse grounds his approach in the work of Szasz (1982) and Flew (1973). In the latter, Boorse says, we find a 'defence . . . of the thesis that physiological medicine should be viewed as the paradigm health discipline' (Boorse, 1982, p. 45, n.2). Examples of authors who use the paradigm form of the likeness argument are Brown (1985, p. 556), who argues from forms of abnormality in physical illness to those in behaviours or experiences (concluding that the likenesses are not present); and Fulford (1989, p. 110) who announces that he will argue from 'chorea, ataxia and paralysis' via 'pain' to mental illness. A number of authors also use the paradigm form of the argument to assess claims of illness status for specific conditions. Claridge (1992) models schizophrenia on hypertension; Ausubel (1967, pp. 261–2) argues from the maladaptions and maladjustments in physical disease to the same features in personality disorder, concluding that it too is a disease.

In the second main form of the likeness argument, the generic approach, 'a generic concept of disease is elicited by abstraction from the concept of bodily disease, and mental disease is then taken to be a species falling under that genus' (Donagan, 1978, p. 42). The abstraction Donagan mentions involves eliciting a concept of disease that does not rely upon anything physical for its realization. Culver and Gert (1982, p. 65), for example believe that 'the same criteria apply to mental conditions as to physical conditions' when it comes to deciding whether or not they are maladies. They hold that 'there is no fundamental difference in kind between physical and mental maladies' (p. 91). They say their definition of malady reflects this by containing 'no reference to bodily (biochemical or physiological) states or processes' (p. 86). It is in virtue of this impartiality between the physical and mental that their approach is generic. A number of other authors also recruit the generic form of the likeness argument, for example Fulford (1989, p. 141), Whitbeck (1981, p. 615), and Brody (1985, pp. 250–1).

As Donagan's account signals, however, the differences between the paradigm and generic accounts seem to be ones of emphasis, and they are quite compatible. The generic concept starts as an abstraction from the concept of bodily disease: that is to say the physical illnesses are, as in the paradigm version, the starting point. And Boorse notes that his paradigm analysis of health 'though derived from physiology, shows no obvious partiality to body over mind. Physical health is simply the special case obtained by focusing on the functions of the physiological processes. Mental health, then, would be the special case obtained by focusing on the functions of the mental processes . . .' (Boorse, 1982, p. 31).

And this is to say that a generic concept (showing 'no obvious partiality to body over mind') is used in the paradigm argument to make the extension from the physical ('bodily') to the mental possible.

The likeness argument and the dispute about the reality of mental illness

The likeness argument is supposed to answer—one way or the other—the radical questions identified before. Notwithstanding it is generally the case that the dispute about what the answer to them should be continues: Szasz has not been silenced (2001, 2002), and Boorse and Fulford still do not agree with one another (cf. Boorse, 1997 and Fulford, 2001). No one version of the argument dominates the field. In this sense, the likeness argument seems to have failed those who set out to use it.

The question is why it has failed, and whether this is a problem lying in the very nature of the argument itself, or some less drastic failure, perhaps in its application. A number of writers have offered reasons why particular versions of the likeness argument have failed to bring agreement to the field (cf. Champlin's response to Szasz, 1989; Fulford's account of Kendell and Szasz, 1989, pp. 5–7). What is notable with these writers, however, is that while they demonstrate problems with opponents' usage of the argument, they stop short of criticizing the argument itself.[1]

An example is Fulford's interesting account of the dispute about whether there is any such thing as mental illness between Szasz and Kendell (1989, pp. 5–7). Though Szasz and Kendell both recruit a paradigm likeness argument, Fulford notices that each calls upon different features of his chosen paradigm (physical illness) in order to prove his case. This explains, as Fulford neatly points out, why despite the fact that both use the likeness argument, they manage to reach opposite conclusions. As a result, neither can necessarily hope to convince the other, or anyone else for that matter, and the radical question goes unresolved. This clearly represents a problem in using the paradigm version of the likeness argument, which is one of Fulford's principal points. However, it turns out that Fulford is not objecting to the use of the likeness argument as such, for he too uses it (in both its forms) abstracting (as Donagan would say) a generic concept of illness (action failure) from paradigmatic physical examples of illness, and employing that to try and resolve the question of whether mental illness exists, by showing that action failure defines illness, and is a principal feature of conditions such as schizophrenia and alcoholism.

The objections to the likeness argument, which will be discussed in this chapter, are not of the kind Fulford raises, but to the form the argument takes.

It will be suggested that two of the assumptions the likeness argument makes to try and ensure it resolves the radical questions about mental illness and about particular claimed mental illnesses are mistaken. If this suggestion is right, there must be some doubt about the capacity of the likeness argument to demonstrate that any particular condition is an illness, or to clinch disputes about the reality of mental illness. Its failure to do so to this point will not be accidental, but inevitable.

Two assumptions of the likeness argument

The two assumptions of the likeness argument in question are related to the ability of the likeness argument to resolve disputes about the reality or existence of mental illness. In both the generic and the paradigm modes of the likeness argument the target is to establish whether a condition such as schizophrenia is an illness or not. If the likeness argument is to resolve this dispute two things must, I think, be taken to be the case:

1. that there are features of human conditions such as schizophrenia, which decide what category, or kind, these conditions are a member of, and
2. that, with respect to the presence or absence of these features, a condition such as schizophrenia is describable independent of the category it is assigned to.

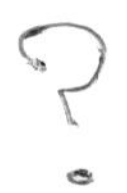

Making the first assumption enables those who use the likeness argument to conclude that, given some condition has the features of illness, it will be an illness, and that further resistance to this conclusion will be futile. So, given that schizophrenia is (to take Boorse's account for a moment) a dysfunction, it will follow that schizophrenia is of the same kind or category as other dysfunctions (in Boorse's conceptualization, it will be a disease; for the full definition see Boorse, 1977, p. 562, or 1997, pp. 7–8). Clearly, once one has made this assumption it would be absurd to continue to claim that mental illnesses do not exist, or that schizophrenia is not an illness, when it has been found that schizophrenia meets the criterion or criteria for being an illness.

Making the second assumption enables those who use the likeness argument to expect agreement that the condition in question has—or has not—the features which, under the first assumption, determine whether it is an illness. Taking Boorse's account again, the second assumption is that those engaged in the dispute about whether mental illness exists or about whether schizophrenia is an illness, will be able to agree whether or not, say, schizophrenia is a dysfunction. The only condition placed on this agreement is that it should be possible without a prior agreement on whether schizophrenia is or is not an illness.

Together, these two assumptions will ensure that the likeness argument is capable of resolving the questions does mental illness exist and/or is *X* an illness. The first assumption hands the question of classification over to the likenesses to sort out, and the second assumption makes sure that the existence of these likenesses is not itself part and parcel of the answer to these questions. Taken together, these two assumptions remove from the issue the role of human agency. If the assumptions of the likeness argument are correct, answering the question whether conditions such as schizophrenia, ADHD, or alcoholism are illnesses is by no means anything to do with the way we happen to think about, conceptualize, or perceive these conditions.

It is these two assumptions and their implication that the existence of mental illness is not down to human agency, that this book questions, by advancing a weak and a strong objection to them. The weak objection is weak in the sense of being less fundamental. In fact the likeness argument can adapt to it, and plausibly come out a better argument for doing so. It questions the first assumption of the likeness argument. The strong objection is strong in the sense of being more fundamental: it altogether undermines both assumptions of the likeness argument. Furthermore, it will be argued that it can be made to stick. Both objections focus on the issue of the role of human agency in answering the question whether mental illness exists or, in the case of specific conditions, whether they are or are not illnesses. The question is how we are to understand this role: the argument put forward here is that it is the sort of role that is implied by the strong objection that is the correct one.

2.3 The weak objection

The objection

The weak objection starts from the observation that, while it may be true that so-called mental illnesses, on the one hand, and physical or bodily illnesses, on the other, have much in common, it is also true that they have many differences. This is true even among physical illnesses, where, for example, some do and some do not lead to raised temperatures. The weak objection does not deny that there are similarities between physical illnesses and mental illnesses; for instance cancer, pneumonia, schizophrenia, and mood disorders may all exhibit dysfunctions. None the less, the weak objection starts from the equally obvious differences, for example that one tends to associate mental illness with behaviours and beliefs, whereas one associates physical illness with physical sufferings—pains, and so on.

The weak objection asks why the similarities should be taken to bring these conditions into a single category, when the differences do not have the effect of putting them in different ones. The point is made by Svensson in his careful consideration of the concept of mental illness (Svensson, 1990). Svensson argues that Szasz's view is not refuted by the likenesses (analogies) appealed to by Margolis (1980), Macklin (1981), or Ausubel (1967).

> This pointing out of analogies between mental disturbances and physical diseases is of course plausible, but only if we have already made up our mind

> to regard and interpret mental problems as diseases. If we have not made up our minds to do this we should certainly ask: In what important respects do mental problems show *dissimilarities* to physical diseases? (p. 46, Svensson's emphasis).

An answer available to a proponent of the likeness argument seems to be that the differences are real enough, but that it is the similarities that count. However, an objector can point out that counting is not one of the features of a condition, but is rather a decision taken by humans with respect to these features, a meaning or importance granted to them. This seems to be contrary to the first assumption, which insists that it is the features that decide which category things fall into, rather than a matter of human interpretation (human agency). It is not possible for the proponent of the likeness argument to reply that the similarities speak for themselves, for if they do, then the same should be true of the differences. The weak objection, then, is that the likeness argument actually relies on a human decision to interpret, or see, the likenesses as having significance.

The first assumption then is not strictly true, the objector argues, and in a damaging way: Similarities to physical illnesses cannot, on their own, bring so-called mental illnesses into the illness category. This is a damaging problem for the likeness argument as it will not be able to resolve the dispute it sets out to resolve if it has to rely on agreed interpretations regarding the meaning of likenesses among the disputants. Nor, as Svensson says, is there any prior reason why the disputants should focus only on similarities.

The plausibility of the weak objection, and responses to it

At least one point weighs heavily in favour of the weak objection. Contrary to the idea that likenesses on their own bring things into categories, we can see two things as having similarities without drawing the conclusion that they are of the same kind. That classical guitars and xylophones are both instruments made of wood does not entail that they are the same sort of instrument, e.g. both percussion instruments. Many things are of the same colour—snow and snow geese, for example. But it does not follow that both are of the same category (unless the category is 'white things' that is). What seems required to get from the likenesses between things to their identity as members of a kind, is an agreement about significance.

An initial response on behalf of the likeness argument might be to appeal to the special relationship that some features of things may have with the category into which those things are placed. This response notes that we can distinguish between features that are more or less incidental in this respect and those that are defining, or perhaps essential. Captain Pugwash's pirate ship flies a skull-and-crossbones flag, but that is not what makes *The Black Pig* a privateer—she is as much a pirate ship when she runs up the white flag. Pneumonia involves a feeling of being ill, but this may be incidental to the category of the thing pneumonia is. Hence, if, far from feeling ill, hypomania is a state of 'ebulliance, boundless optimism, euphoria and self-confidence' (Champlin, 1989, p. 27) that will not matter. On the other hand, pneumonia's being a dysfunction of some kind may be regarded as defining, so it will matter whether or not mania is also a dysfunction. Nor, it may be argued, need the importance of these features rely on some form of human decision or stipulation—the very thing the likeness argument seeks to avoid. This response supports the first assumption of the likeness argument, by suggesting that the features of things may, after all, be what are decisive when it comes to their categorization.

The question is then whether this response receives any support: is it reasonable to assume that notions such as illness stand in a one-to-one relation with a set of features? I shall look at two considerations which suggest that this is an unreasonable thing to expect to be true in the case of illness. The first of these arises from the work of psychologists, and is the claim that this presupposition represents an empirically unrealistic view of actual concept formation. The second consideration is that, given the range of conditions we call illnesses, it is highly unlikely that any such feature or set of features exists. However, I shall suggest that the likeness argument can recruit some resources to resist these reasons for thinking that there can be no one-to-one relationship between the notion of illness and a set of features.

Concept formation

The first reason for thinking that this neat one-to-one relationship does not exist comes from the data that psychologists have gathered concerning concept formation. Of particular relevance to us here is the work of Eleanor Rosch (1977). She brings evidence apparently to bear against the idea that concepts are defined in terms of a list of essential features (an idea sometimes referred to as the classical view). In the way we normally conceptualize things, Rosch says, people are often unable to give anything like a defining set of characteristics (Keil, 1992, p. 27). In fact there is no one-to-one relationship between their features and the category they fall into. She says that the classical view ignores the evidence that many concepts have what she calls internal structure. To take an example, the concept 'bird' might be formed around the regularly co-appearing attributes of feathers, wings, and beaks. (Rosch notes that these co-occur at better than chance rates in reality and that this is why the concept forms around them.) However, not all birds have all these features, and so some birds will be regarded as prototypical of the category (sparrows, blackbirds, and such like) while others (maybe penguins) will be regarded as more marginal. This prototypicality and comparative marginality constitutes the internal structure of the category. Rosch believes that the classical view of concepts fails to reflect this internal structure. It does so because it supposes that every member of the category will have all the features that mark the category out—all will be equally prototypical (in Rosch's language). However, Rosch argues this is a mistake. And so, if Rosch is right, the claim that there is a special relation between the defining features of a thing and its membership in categories would be a mistake too. Generally speaking, Rosch would say, the evidence suggests such special one-to-one relationships do not exist. The likeness argument certainly cannot presuppose that the concept of illness will have such an essence.

Rosch's argument is also important from our point of view, because it looks as though the weak objection to the likeness argument can recruit her point to back up its claim that human decisions have to be made to interpret the meaning of features. In some cases it seems that something can be a bird but not have a feature that a prototypical bird has. Penguins are birds, despite the absence of feathers. They may be marginal birds, in terms of the structure of the category bird, but they are said to be birds none the less. On the other hand, some features such as beaks are found in creatures that are not included in the category bird (the octopus and the duck-billed platypus spring to mind). Though they have a common feature of birds, they are not said to be birds, not even marginal birds. How is this to be explained? Clearly having some of the features prototypical birds have is sometimes enough, and sometimes not. Some decision seems to be required relating to whether the features that penguins and octopuses have will count. Humans seem to have to decide whether the fact that the octopus has a beak will make it a bird, and whether the fact that the penguin does not have feathers mean it isn't a bird. Rosch's approach seems to create the necessity for human interpretation of the features of the world and their role in classification. Applying the argument to say ADHD, it may be said that it is a dysfunction, and that this does make it an illness even though the person who has ADHD does not suffer physical pain. An interpretation is clearly part of this picture.

The weak objection could perhaps, then, recruit Rosch's views for its own purposes. But before we accept this, we need to determine whether Rosch's claims about concepts are right. They have been subject to some criticism. Among those who have criticized aspects of Rosch's work is Frank Keil (1992). Keil points out that the data Rosch uses to support her arguments against the classical view of concepts is not in fact inconsistent with it. Though it may lend support to her claim that concepts are structured around prototypes, it can equally be interpreted to support the classical view. For example, among the data underlying her conclusions were experiments relating to how quickly people identified examples of certain kinds, and how likely people were to name particular examples when asked to give a member of a certain kind. Rosch found that people more quickly identify say sparrows than penguins as examples of the kind bird, or were more likely to give sparrow than penguin as an example of a bird. However, Keil reports evidence that similar effects can be derived in examples in which a classical account of concepts looks entirely apposite. Armstrong *et al.* (1983) tested people on examples of the concept 'odd number' and found people regarded some odd numbers as more typical than others. If, Keil argues, a category easy enough to define classically can give rise to 'internal structure' then we cannot infer a non-classical conceptualization from the presence of internal structure (1992, pp. 29–30). More generally, Keil says that psychologists have been too hasty to jump from their empirical data to conclusions about concepts (p. 27).

If we apply this to the concept illness, it can be argued that even if it were shown that the concept illness has an internal structure of the kind Rosch believes other concepts to have, it does not follow that it has no defining set of features. If this is true, it does not after all help the weak objection to the likeness argument to appeal to this aspect of Rosch's work. The idea that concepts may have some form of classical unity or essence survives Rosch's empirical data.

The variability of illnesses

But it may be that there is another sort of reason for rejecting the classical view. That is that given the range of conditions we call illnesses, it is highly unlikely that any feature or set of features exists that all illnesses would have. At first sight this seems reasonably persuasive. However, within philosophy there is still strong support for the idea that the concept illness has unity such that it can be defined in classical, i.e. necessary and sufficient (or at least necessary) terms, and a parallel rejection of an alternative family resemblance account (e.g. Fulford, 1989, p. 134; Brody, 1985, p. 250). Moreover, it may be perfectly reasonable and legitimate to seek to unify a concept around one or two defining features; Boorse argues, for example, that this is required to place limits around the application of a concept (1977, p. 545).

To sum up the argument so far: Rosch's objection to the classical view of concepts turns out to be questionable. And philosophically speaking, the idea that there are clear fixed lists of features of things that decide into which category they should be placed retains support. We have so far no reason to abandon the idea that illness is a classically structured concept. So the assumption that it is the features of illnesses that decide for us whether schizophrenia is an illness, to take an example—the first assumption of the likeness argument—has so far survived attempts to show it is incorrect.

The bi-determination of concepts

However, this is not sufficient to meet the nub of weak objection. Even if concepts, including the concept of illness, are classically structured, it does not follow that human agency is not involved. Rosch, for example, suggests that human concepts reflect real-world greater-than-chance co-occurrences of features (such as, in the case of birds, beaks, feathers, and wings). If these features determine what our concepts are and determine what counts as an example of a particular concept, then it would appear, at first sight, that the first assumption is supported. However, she also says that while the principles of category formation are universal the categories that are formed and their content are not (Rosch, 1977, pp. 39–40). Even though concepts form around real world correlations, she points out that in different cultures interest in the attributes of the world and their correlations may vary (p. 39). The concepts we have reflect something other than such natural correlations. We are not interested in all features of the world, she suggests, and so do not necessarily take notice of some correlations. So our concepts at least in part reflect us. She also notes how those who have a specialist knowledge in a certain field may be aware of different features of things than are others who have only a lay knowledge in that particular area. To extrapolate that to psychiatry, it may be that being a psychiatrist enables one to see correlating and defining features invisible to others.

The points I have just taken from Rosch reflect perhaps the underlying and most important point in the weak objection, namely the significance of what Bellaimey calls the bi-directional determination of concepts (Bellaimey, 1990). These two directions of determination are the input of the things themselves, that is to say their own features; and the input of human decision making, values, and interests. In accounts of the concept of illness, for example, it is commonly argued that the concept illness represents to some degree a value judgement. If this were the case, then what falls into the category represents in part the making of this judgement—which is a human decision, based upon human interests. The first assumption would fail because the features of a human condition alone would not be enough to determine its category.

Can the likeness argument survive this point, or does it have to give way? It depends on how one believes the human interests and values operate. One way of rescuing, and ultimately strengthening, the likeness argument might be to show that it can accommodate the role of human values and interests, without giving up the first assumption. A route to showing this is provided by Renford Bambrough's account of Wittgenstein's family resemblance theory of concepts (Bambrough, 1970). Bambrough argues that a system of classification—that is to say the range of categories into which things may be classified—represents the interests of a particular group of people, living in a particular way, in particular historical, social, and environmental circumstances. What these interests do is to serve as a basis for a range of categories, and for picking out the particular features of things. These features then play the role of placing things into categories.

Bambrough illustrates the point. He imagines an island community reliant upon wood for building its boats and houses, which divides trees up into categories such as 'boat building trees' and 'house building trees'. These categories, he supposes, would be constituted quite differently to those that visiting Western botanists have developed, such as 'date palm', 'cedar', and so on. To the Western botanists, a group of trees which the islanders say are all of the same type, might appear to be a hodge-podge of botanically distinct varieties. By the same token, a homogeneous clump in Western botanical eyes may appear to the islanders to be a merely random grouping.

However, this does not undermine the role of likenesses in Bambrough's account, and goes some way to offering qualified support to the first assumption of the likeness argument. For what, according to Bambrough, makes some individual tree a member of a class (be it a Western or an Island class) is the objective features of the tree, that the classification system causes to be picked out. To fill out Bambrough's example, we might imagine that boat building trees are those that are objectively big enough to build boats, but in which the wood is still pliable enough to be moulded into shape. On the other hand, house building trees would be more rigid, and so on. Likewise, Western botany has picked out certain defining features—or patterns of features—of date palms and cedars.

Relating all this to the likeness argument, the point is that the role of human decisions, interests, and values is taken up in the development of a system of classification of human conditions, including the distinction of conditions into illnesses and non-illnesses. But once that system is developed, the classification takes on a life of its own, reliant on the similarities the system of classification caused to be picked out. Perhaps, at some point in the past, the negative impact certain conditions have upon human lives led to the development of a category of 'illness' for them. However, since then, so the argument would go, we have found among illnesses shared features that characterize them. These might represent the essences that Keil argues may be present within concepts, and an example of such an essence might be Boorse's notion of dysfunction. True, then, there is a role for human values and interests; but it is in the background. There is a sense in which the likeness argument relies distantly upon its existence, but not after all damagingly so. Moreover, as the years pass, the original interests and values enshrined in a system of classification may cease to be operative in society more generally, while the system itself continues (as indeed would seem to have to be the case with the Western botanical classifications, supposing they originate in human values and interests).

Bambrough's approach offers qualified but distinct support for the first assumption of the likeness argument. And Bambrough's approach is reflected in some more recent work in the psychology of concept formation. To recap and summarize: that assumption states that human conditions such as schizophrenia are illnesses—or are not—in virtue of their features. The weak objection states that these features are not enough: we should not forget the role of human decisions and interests. However, these may play a rather background role, leaving the features of categories to determine things in practice. This is a significant concession to the likeness argument, and one that I think plausibly strengthens it by showing how to take into account the widely acknowledged role of values in categorizations such as illness without giving up the first assumption.

2.4 The strong objection to the likeness argument

This section explores what I call the strong objection to the likeness argument. The weak objection to the likeness argument focused on the first assumption of the likeness argument, which is that it is the features of things that determine of what kind they are. The strong objection takes exception to the second assumption. The second assumption is that the features of human conditions such as schizophrenia are describable independently of the category the conditions are part of. As was indicated earlier, this assumption is necessary to the likeness argument, which relies on agreement over what the features of human conditions are. Bambrough signals this by talking about the objectivity of the similarities that are picked out within systems of classification. Likewise, Rosch talks of attributes that correlate in the real world. In setting out the second assumption, objectivity is not, however, demanded: the agreement over description of the features needs only to be independent of the dispute the existence of those features is intended to resolve.

The strong objection, in short, is that the description of the features does not meet this requirement. Three examples will be used to advance and explain the strong objection. The first example concerns the features of alcoholism, the second ADHD, and the third schizophrenia. In all three cases the aim will be to show that the description of the features of each is part and parcel of its category membership. Things come to be categorized by humans, and in the light of that they take on features associated with that kind of thing. The classification or category into which things fall, the features they are perceived to have, and the work of human agency are all closely connected in the case of illness.

Alcoholism

Scientists have long been engaged in the search for evidence of links between so-called mental illnesses and people's physical constitution. Karl Jaspers' account of the diagnostic schema of mental illnesses in the early twentieth century reflects this. He notes that it was believed that the major psychoses (which were taken to be epilepsy, schizophrenia, and manic depressive disease) would prove to have 'a somatic base'. They would then be categorized with somatic illnesses that caused psychic disturbances (such as infections and General Paralysis; Jaspers, 1997 [1913], pp. 605ff). The catecholamine theory of depression of 1965, and the dopamine theory of schizophrenia of the early 70s both hypothesized chemical bases for these diseases (see Healy, 1990, pp. 65–7; Kupfer, 1991). But the idea that some causal link of a physical kind must exist to mental illness can be identified much earlier, in the nineteenth century. The interest in the genetic basis of schizophrenia, for example, is historically more or less contemporary with the idea that those mental conditions we might now put down to schizophrenia should be seen as a medical problem (see Marshall, 1992 and Boyle, 1990, p. 118). From the point of view of the argument of this chapter and the book as a whole, the significance of these views is that they point to the existence of features that are found in physical illnesses, and are plausibly taken to be important evidence for something being an illness. They are just the kind of feature that someone who utilizes the likeness argument might appeal to.

There have been suggestions that alcoholism is related to irregular alpha-rhythms in the brain (Vogel and Propping, 1981) and more recently to craving (Anton, 2001). Vogel and Propping (1981) speculate that 'individuals with irregular alpha-waves experience so much improvement in their state of mind [when they take a drink] that they are more easily conditioned to succumb to alcohol than persons with regular alpha activity' (p. 276). Anton defines craving as: '. . . a state of the brain, created by years of heavy alcohol use, that undermines 'free will' and motivates alcoholics to continue to use alcohol despite irrefutable evidence of harm to themselves or the people close to them' (Anton, 2001, p. 11).

An important neurochemical system underlying craving is the dopamine system, which may mediate memory of the rewarding aspects of alcohol, playing a role in making this memory 'heightened and inappropriate' (Anton, 2001, p. 11) and thus increasing the likelihood of relapse.

However, despite their claims, neither Vogel and Propping nor Anton has done enough to make out a decisive case for a causal link. Even supposing that having the irregular alpha rhythms causes a heightened pleasure to be had from drinking alcohol, and that makes conditioning easier, that would not necessarily make it a cause of alcoholism.[2] Whether one wants to repeat that pleasure need be nothing to do with the alpha rhythm patterns that are correlated with excessive drinking. Likewise, the fact that one has inappropriately rosy memories of the times when one was under the influence of alcohol because of the effect of alcohol upon dopamine, does not make dopamine a cause of relapse. The attitude one has to one's past experiences, whether these were distorted or not, need not be affected by dopamine. That one felt good when drinking does not mean one has to want to recapture the feeling. In both cases, the willingness to give in, or the failure to hold out, may be to do with one's moral fortitude. The right question here may be: is one of such strong moral fibre that one can resist such temptations to fall victim to the demon drink. If one is not made of such moral fibre, and one gives in, one is not ill. One is simply morally weak and easily led by certain pleasures or the memory of certain pleasures off the straight and narrow.[3]

The issue here is the interpretation of scientific evidence. A possible interpretation of this evidence in the case of alcoholism shows that it is not a disease after all, but is rather a condition of moral weakness. That is not to say that alcoholism is definitely not a disease; the idea that it is seems at least plausible. However, what is at stake here is whether certain observable or detectable facts can decide, or help decide, the issue, as the likeness argument claims. And when we look closely we see that the facts about the correlation of physical structures and events to alcoholism can be described in two quite different ways, leading to two quite different conclusions about what kind of condition alcoholism is. The detectable and observable features of alcoholism do not determine what description should be given of them.

And on this rock the second assumption of the likeness argument founders. The existence of a resemblance of physical causation between say alcoholism and physical illness proves to rely upon a prior choice to describe alcoholism in one way rather than another. The description one takes to be correct reflects the category into which alcoholism is placed. This is directly contrary to the second assumption: the relevant features of alcoholism do not, contrary to what it demands, exist independently of the category into which alcoholism is placed.

Attention deficit hyperactivity disorder

There are claims for many mental illnesses that they have a genetic basis. This has been said of alcoholism and of schizophrenia. But for the purposes of the argument here, I will consider a different case, that of ADHD. Accardo and Blondis (2000) suggest that ADHD behaviours are a well enough defined pattern to consider seriously that it is caused by some genetic mutation. They say 'one cannot fail to notice how commonly symptoms of inattention, impulsivity, and hyperactivity occur in a various combinations within the clinical descriptions of most behavioral phenotypes being identified' (p. 8). In the light of this, they compare ADHD behaviours with Smith–Magenis syndrome (SMS). SMS appears in children, and is constituted by a similarly well defined behavioural pattern: 'Self-hugging ('spasmodic upper-body squeeze'), onychotillomania (pulling out of fingernails and toenails), [and] polyembolokoilomania (insertion of foreign bodies into bodily orifices)' (p. 8). 'Carefully focussed' genetic research relating to these behaviours has revealed a 'tiny deletion that causes their appearance (17p11.2)' (p. 8). Their point is that this suggests we should not give up the search for a genetic basis for ADHD behaviours.

Accardo and Blondis's case can be developed into a challenge to the strong objection to the likeness argument—though this is not the way they actually do develop their argument, and is my development rather than theirs. If a genetic deletion were discovered that correlated with the behavioural triad of inattention, impulsivity, and hyperactivity in the way the deletion at 17p11.2 correlates with the behaviours of SMS (i.e. pretty much one-to-one) would that not in effect be a discovery of a causal connection? And does not the possibility of such a discovery support the second assumption of the likeness argument? The argument would be that the discovery proves or irresistibly suggests a causal account—it is not the result of categorization, but rather may play a part in deciding that ADHD behaviours are to be explained as an illness (i.e. by ADHD).

However, in the case of ADHD behaviours, the proponent of the strong objection can respond in a way that mirrors the response in the case of alcoholism. It can be argued that the failure to pay attention reflects something other than causal and ultimately physical forces. Supporting this line of argument is Carl Elliott's description of a friend of his (he calls him Grady) who has been diagnosed as an adult with ADHD. Elliott writes:

> Once he became familiar with the signs and symptoms of ADHD, he found it harder and harder to tolerate things that seemed symptomatic of his condition: forgetting to pick up groceries on the way home, taking a long time to leave the house every morning, failing to clean up his office or apartment. Before the diagnosis these just seemed like permanent features of his character, but afterward he found himself saying, 'Damn, it took me forty-five minutes to get out of the house today. Plus I zoned out at the meeting today. . . .' He says it became easier to see his habits as personal failures, and harder to see them as a natural reaction to his circumstances. (p. 256)

For Grady, tendencies in his behaviour take on the nature of a challenge: they present Grady with a problem that he conceives as his personal responsibility to overcome. If Grady zones out in a meeting or gets distracted while getting ready for work in the morning it can be said that he has failed in this personal responsibility. Someone can plausibly argue that this suggests that even though Grady may have a clear behavioural pattern of distractibility, what matters is his failure or otherwise to overcome this.

Two arguments can be put up against this claim: the first is that Grady is fooling himself—contrary to what he thinks, he actually does not have any choice. But this argument can be put aside. What I am relying on here is not the experience or belief of Grady about himself, but the alternative conceptualization that his understanding of his condition represents. The second argument against the claim that Grady's story undermines the notion of causality is more fundamental. It is that genes may play a causal role without determining behaviour. They can predispose or render someone susceptible to behaviours of certain kinds, and this is what is meant by causality in the case of genes and behaviour. This indeed appears to be backed up by current genetic studies. Summarizing these, Cook (2000, p. 22) writes that: 'evidence exists that genetic factors contribute to susceptibility to ADHD. With two independent replications, it appears that the dopamine transporter locus influences ADHD expression.'

Grady's experience, it might be said, is a good example of how such susceptibilities or predispositions may appear—i.e. as a personal challenge.

The problem with this second more fundamental argument, as far as the proponent of the likeness argument is concerned, is that the strong objection can embrace it. It can do so by questioning what is meant by predisposition. Suppose that what was meant was that those who have the genetic deletion are more likely to behave in the way described as ADHD (and similarly with claims about alcoholism and genetic predisposition). This does not prove anything about causality. The question is what are we to conceive of as characterizing the role of the genes in the individual's behaviour. It may be that they are conceived in terms of character weaknesses.

It might be argued that in children, which is where ADHD is usually diagnosed, this thesis about predisposition is weaker. The argument might be that in the case of children, where character has not yet been formed, self-awareness is less developed, and moral codes less well internalized, talk of personal challenge or personal failing is misplaced and a causal account is more plausible. But it is not clear that this argument works. If it is argued that in children character is less developed, and this explains the impact of the genes upon their behaviour, then the focus is still on character rather than causality. It is just acknowledged that we should expect less of a child's character faced by temptations to do something more fun than study, for example. This is something we generally accept about children. If children want more sweets than is good for them that is not necessarily a reason for thinking that their behaviour is determined by their genes. Rather, we may say that such wants are typical of the desires and value structures of the immature. We do not necessarily blame the child for this—immaturity is a characteristic of most children. But nor do we necessarily need to impute anything such as genetic causation.

The issues turn out to revolve around questions of where and how we focus. The genetic causal (or predisposal) story implicit in ADHD proves to be part and parcel of one way of looking at what is going on. The mere presence of genetic correlations with inattentive, impulsive, and hyperactive behaviour does not determine that we must give an account of the behaviour in illness terms, i.e. in terms of ADHD. If we opt for the causal account, we show we are already thinking in illness terms. If ADHD is our conceptualization of what is going on, then this reveals how we are thinking.

Schizophrenia[4]

Alcoholism and ADHD may be eccentric cases. Certainly, as far as illness classification is concerned, both seem to be borderline cases. Psychiatrists may be quite happy to admit that alcoholism and ADHD are not illnesses, or that perception of the sort of thing they are is variable, changing with the way people think of them. Schizophrenia seems to be a central case. We may turn our attention here to the notion that schizophrenia, and other major psychoses, are dysfunctions of the mind (cf. Boorse, 1982; Wakefield, 1992a (p. 375), b (p. 246)) and in particular to the belief that it results from a malfunction of its mechanisms of self-monitoring and self-awareness (Frith, 1992). (Note that ADHD is also described in functional terms, by Barkley (1997) for example.)

One reason for thinking that people have schizophrenia is that they often believe odd or bizarre things about others and themselves. People believe that others can read their thoughts, that aliens are controlling their actions, that they are being communicated with by famous people, or that their actions somehow affect world events (Frith, 1992, pp. 4–5). It is sometimes argued that holding such beliefs suggests a dysfunction of the mind. Boorse thinks that 'the main function of the perceptual and intellectual processes is to give us knowledge of the world' (Boorse, 1982, p. 42). Most of us, if we have such thoughts at all, may be said to check them against reality, realize they are clearly wrong, and not make them our beliefs. On the dysfunction approach, people with schizophrenia would be unable to do this, as whatever most have that checks such odd thoughts and rejects them, is not working for them.

Is a dysfunction account the correct account to give here? Even though we may be absolutely sure that the person has false beliefs, and that any reasonable person, even if they entertained these beliefs, would soon be persuaded away from them, it is a further step to argue that this is evidence of a dysfunction. It is reasonable to claim that people can check reality, of course. There are all sorts of ways of establishing for ourselves the truth or falsity of statements, be they, to take an example at random, about today's cricket scores, or about whether aliens are controlling one's actions. However, from the fact that we can do this, it does not follow that there is some part of our psychological make up, some aspect of our minds, which has this function. We can also make mistakes about reality, but that need not suggest that there is some part of our mind that plays the part of trying to delude us. Rather than thinking of checking reality in functional terms, we might think of checking reality as a practice that we carry out as carefully or as haphazardly as we wish using socially learned and variable tools. Someone who believes she is being controlled by aliens may be thought of as failing to check reality, checking using the wrong tools, feeling unable or not wanting to check the reality of her particular beliefs. In none of these cases do we have to think of dysfunction.

A relatively recent version of the claim that schizophrenia is a dysfunction is that of Frith (1992). Frith argues, for example, that the thoughts experienced as inserted by schizophrenics are in fact their own thoughts (Frith, 1992, p. 73; see also Szasz, 1996). Frith's explanation of this reported phenomenon is that there is a failure properly to self-monitor (pp. 73ff), which he hypothesizes is an aspect of a wider failure of self-awareness (chapter 7). Because they fail to monitor their actions, such as thinking, schizophrenics confuse their own thinking with having thoughts inserted. Frith believes that the explanation for this breakdown of self-awareness and self-monitoring is to be found in the brain (pp. 84ff, 126ff). Understanding of the causal lesion is at a very early stage, but Frith reports that there is in general a revived interest in the thesis that schizophrenia is 'a disease of the brain' (chapter 2). Recent studies of schizophrenia look at genetic, biochemical, and brain functional factors in trying to sort out why and in what way the brains of schizophrenics are diseased (Keefe and Harvey, 1994). Frith's hypothesis also covers acts which may be reported as controlled by outside forces (1992, pp. 81ff).

The appeal to a brain lesion clearly suggests that Frith believes the failure of self-monitoring is a dysfunction of a brain system that functions to monitor.

But, while the functional account seems plausible, it is clear that it is not forced upon us. There is the possibility that there is an interpretive element to an individual's experience of thought and self. If the self is a concept developed by the individual, influenced by cultural and historical settings, then it can be developed in various ways. Thus, someone who experiences certain thoughts as inserted may be conceived not as having a dysfunction in monitoring, but as being especially sensitive to thoughts that—as we may all experience from time to time—appear to be less obviously the result of active thinking (thoughts that simply 'come into' our heads). This sensitivity may arise in the light of the person's view of what constitutes the self. What, for most, would be interpreted as a thought that simply came unbidden into the mind, might for a person with a different notion of the self be interpreted as someone else's thought inserted into his or her mind.

This implies no dysfunction of monitoring, as it is explained by different conceptualizations of the self, and resulting interpretations of experiences, and not by any failure to self-monitor. As a result, with respect to Frith's belief concerning the brain systems that underlie the supposed function of self-monitoring, these seem now to correlate only with different conceptualizations of the self. But there appears to be no motivation for accounting for these in physical causal terms: differences in conceptualizations are not usually explained in that way, nor indeed regarded as pathological.

It is not being argued here that these alternative, non-functional, accounts of schizophrenia are correct. Rather, as with the non-causal accounts of alcoholism or of ADHD, the point is that alternative descriptions of the scientific facts or observed phenomena are possible. In some of these alternatives, illness-like features disappear. For example, causal features are replaced by the ordinary motivations of human individuals—the reasons for which they act; dysfunctions are replaced by differing interpretations and conceptualizations. The illness-like features reappear when the behaviours in question—the behaviours of alcoholism, ADHD, or aspects of schizophrenia—are described in illness terms. But this is contrary to the second assumption of the likeness argument. The illness-like features of the conditions in question do not appear independently of their classification as illnesses.

The second objection and the first assumption

The second objection also provides a substantial objection to the first assumption of the likeness argument. That first assumption holds that the features of human conditions determine what category they fall into. However, if the very existence of the features in question comes with the categorization, the first assumption must be wrong. It relies upon the idea that one can infer or deduce the kind or category it falls into from some of the features some condition has. But the objection just considered to the second assumption, if right, makes the features a condition (say schizophrenia) is said to have, part and parcel of its categorization. And the implication of this—fundamental for the rest of this book—is that the business of categorizing alcoholism, ADHD, or schizophrenia goes on in some other way; in short it involves a human decision simply to categorize these conditions as illnesses.

2.5 Arguments against the strong objection

I want to consider two, I think potentially strong, attempted rebuttals of the strong objection, and try to understand and perhaps counter or accommodate them. The first objection will be dealt with mostly here and now. But the second, which alleges that my position will lead to irrationality and scepticism, will be discussed and answered only by the rest of the book.

The first attempted rebuttal is that descriptions in terms of illness are as it were forced upon the observer of a severely psychotic person. So, while a counter description in non-illness terms may be coherent, and not altogether implausible, it would hardly occur to one faced with the phenomena in question. For example, in the case of thought insertion in schizophrenia, the argument would be that the idea that the person is ill would be irresistibly suggested by the phenomenon presented, for all that a clever alternative can be thought up with a bit of effort. With ADHD it is often argued that the amazing disruptive energy of some children leaves no doubt that for them at least some form of pathology is implicated.

However, the attempted rebuttal under consideration is not altogether to the point. The idea that illness is irresistibly suggested by the phenomena when they are presented to us is not relevant to the nature of the likeness argument. The strong objection operates where a certain kind of reason—that is to say the presence of sufficient likenesses—is offered for categorizing something as an illness. It does not pretend to operate where something else may be determining the categorization, for example some kind of intuitive response to what one sees.

There is none the less an important insight behind the attempted rebuttal, which is that it can often be difficult to find an at all plausible alternative account of some phenomena, because one account seems so *natural* (a word used here to try and capture the immediacy and irresistibility to which the rebuttal seems to appeal). One writer who takes up a point of this kind specifically in the context of my objections to the likeness argument is Richard Gipps (2003). He says that we should understand the likeness argument in slightly different terms to the ones I have put forward: 'proponents of the illness conception who deploy the likeness argument are . . . perhaps better understood as attempting to remind us of what they believe we tacitly already know' (Gipps, 2003, p. 256).

So, according to Gipps, the person who uses the likeness argument is not trying to convince others. The likeness argument is not an attempt to make everyone think the same way about it by sheer force of reason; rather the whole argument presupposes a sort of community of agreement in the first place. He is saying that the use of the likeness argument reveals a pretheoretical (p. 257) belief that schizophrenia (to take an example) is an illness.

I would defend my account of the likeness argument, however. It seems to me that my account of what it aims to try and do is truer to what its proponents say it aims to try and do than Gipps' account of it. But Gipps' ideas are none the less important. In particular, he seems to me to be have made an important observation about the possible source of the feeling that to call something like schizophrenia an illness is natural. If he is right, then the naturalness of the idea that there are such things as mental illnesses seems to arise because it is unquestioned (rather than being unquestioned because it's natural). Gipps suggests, in fact, that it is part and parcel of our responses to behaviours such as those of schizophrenics. Part of our experience of the behaviour of the schizophrenic is an experience that they are ill.

However, that something seems natural or pretheoretical in the sense Gipps seems to have in mind need not be taken to be the final word on the matter. The idea that the heart is a pump seems, likewise, a perfectly natural idea, one which appears irresistibly suggested by what the heart does. But the machine model of the heart, it can be argued, is based upon a deeper acceptance that the body as a whole is a machine (Pickering, 1999, pp. 368–70; and see Chapter 5 in this book). Yet this is a view with a historical starting point, which holds sway now only after many years of dispute with alternatives, and may yet have challenges to meet. So, while it may well be the case that we do (generally) respond to schizophrenia as an illness, and while it may well be the case that this response is pretheoretical, it does not follow that it is immune to questioning. At this point, the likeness argument—and hence my objections to it—may reappear.

The second attempted rebuttal of the strong objection might be expressed as follows: 'There is an important ambiguity in your argument. You have spoken of the categorization of alcoholism and of schizophrenia. And you have mentioned the "bi-directional determination of concepts". But categorization is ambivalent between something determined by the conditions themselves, because of their features for example (as the likeness argument holds), and something determined by a categorizer. Your strong objection clearly rests upon an assumption that places you in the second camp. Moreover, it implies, absurdly, that the features things have is determined by how humans categorise them.'

This is potentially a potent objection. And, of course, it would be absurd to claim, for example, that a genetic correlation in ADHD could be produced by simply calling it an illness—or removed by calling it something else. However, this is not the claim made in this chapter.

The claim I am making is that categorizing alcoholism, ADHD, and schizophrenia as illnesses brings with it a description of these conditions in which the features of illness appear. But this is not the same as saying that any description at all is possible. The observed neurochemical correlation hypothesized in the case of alcoholism is what is described: the description of the correlation may be a causal one, or the correlation may be described as a source of moral temptation. The same point arises in the case of hypothesized genetic correlations in the case of ADHD. However, it is the description of the correlation in causal terms, and not the correlation itself, which is the product of the categorization. If no such correlation is to be found, calling alcoholism an illness or categorizing behaviours as ADHD will not create it.

It is, however, true that the belief that some condition is an illness can lead to a research programme aimed at finding certain kinds of correlation. The search for the neurochemical correlates of many conditions has been inspired by recent developments in our knowledge of the neurochemistry of the human brain (Frith, 1992, chapter 2), by developments in neuroimaging techniques (in the case of ADHD for example) and by developments in genetics (as for example in Smith–Magenis syndrome). The question here is only whether, if discovered, neurochemical abnormalities, or genetic deletions, would force a categorization of conditions correlated to them as illnesses. The argument is only that if a research programme were to find a correlation of that kind, this would not necessarily decide the matter of classification.

Lurking behind the objection may be a further important thought, however. And that is that the rejection of the likeness argument seems to introduce an unacceptable element of contingency into the way important questions about the categorization of schizophrenia and alcoholism are answered. There is some truth in this charge. It is true, that is to say, that in this book the appeal to neurochemical correlations described causally, or to descriptions of the mind in terms of dysfunctions, are taken to be historically contingent—reflecting current research programmes, beliefs and technologies rather than truths of nature or biology.

Loughlin (2003) holds that my approach is in danger of falling into a radical sort of scepticism in which our attempts to understand the world are always undermined by our various conceptual schema (e.g. because these schema are limited by our time and place). For example, I argue that in descriptions of alcoholism and schizophrenia there is an interpretative element. This element is in part constituted by the conceptual alternatives (illness, non-illness) we bring to our descriptions. The way I construe the presence of these concepts is such that, or at least seems to be such that it prevents us coming to any useful or penetrating conclusion about what sort of things schizophrenia and alcoholism really are. We can never get our conceptually tinted glasses off and see the world in the pure light of the sun.

But, to the extent that my approach does suggest the sort of scepticism that Loughlin mentions, it is not the arguments advanced in this book against the likeness argument that should be identified as the problem. The likeness argument relies upon the contingently selected features of likeness to decide the dispute about the reality of mental illness. It presents itself, however, as getting beyond these contingencies, and resolving, or at least as being capable of resolving, the dispute about the reality of mental illness. The objections raised to the likeness argument in this chapter are designed to show the insecurity of the widely shared belief in the capacity of the likeness argument to get beyond such contingencies.

None the less, I think Loughlin's comments are well taken. I would not want to embrace the scepticism he describes, as he rightly observes (p. 262). But as will become increasingly apparent in what follows in the rest of the book, I sail very close to the sceptical wind on this one. So I shall constantly have to come back to Loughlin's point.

In this chapter, I seek to avoid scepticism by saying that the interpretations that arise within the conceptual schema of scientists, for example, are supposed to be *of* the scientific facts about alcoholism and schizophrenia, e.g. of the accepted facts of brain chemistry and so on. These facts constitute important insights into the nature of the brain and its workings, albeit they may be based upon a historically limited set of conceptual resources. It's what we make of these insights that is at stake, I believe, in the debate about the reality and nature of mental illness.

Conclusions

The likeness argument dominates the dispute over the reality of mental illness. As a matter of fact, no one has yet produced a version of it which achieves what it aims and claims to be able to achieve, namely to answer the question whether or not conditions such as schizophrenia really are illnesses or not. Disputes continue on all sides about which likenesses and differences are to count, and what they are to count for.

I have argued that the likeness argument cannot close these disputes, because two of the assumptions it relies upon to do so do not stand up to scrutiny. In particular, the idea that the features that should decide the issue (as the first assumption states), are describable independently of views about the issue (as the second assumption states), is false. They are not; and so the likeness argument must fail.

The nature of the failure is, however, instructive. The likeness argument takes it for granted that the radical questions are about what we may observe or discover. Its failure is precisely on this point. Human agency is involved in the categorization of patterns of behaviour as illnesses such as ADHD, alcoholism, or schizophrenia. The rest of this book seeks to work out a conception of how this human role in creating mental illnesses might be understood in greater depth. How do the radical questions—and the various answers given to them—look if we accept that in some sense the answer to the questions lie with human decision, or human agency?

In the second chapter of this part, I propose to turn initially to what I take to be the fundamental article of faith of those who use the likeness argument: it is a third assumption, if you like, of the argument. The argument assumes that it is *possible* that some things could be mental illnesses, and that the difficulty is to establish or discover whether anything is. This presumes that the concept mental illness *makes sense*. Questions about whether or not the notion of mental illness does make sense will lead us to arguments about how coherent the concept is, and a quite different approach to answering the radical questions.

Endnotes

1 But see Champlin (1996). I would like to thank one of the anonymous referees of Pickering (2003) for drawing my attention to this article.
2 Radden (1985, p. 32) argues a similar point at a more general level.
3 A psycho-analytic approach of a Freudian, Jungian, or Adlerian kind might give yet another description. This would involve seeking meaning, though not the moral meaning I have described, in the events, rather than causes. See Healy (1990, p. 58).
4 For a discussion with some parallels to what follows, see Boyle (1990, p. 169).

3 The categorical argument

3.1 Mental illness a classificatory concept

In this chapter, we begin to look at a different way of answering the radical questions about mental illness; different, that is, from the likeness argument, which was presented and criticized in the last chapter.

We have argued that the likeness argument has to be rejected. It has to be rejected because some of its fundamental assumptions are faulty. The likeness argument rests upon the belief that we can find out whether something is or is not a mental illness by relying on its features to tell us. People do not make such categorizing decisions, they are made for humans without human agency. If a condition such as ADHD, to take an example, has the features that characterize illnesses, the likeness argument says, it is an illness. But the arguments of the first part of the book suggest that whether ADHD has features that are like those of other illnesses is part and parcel of its categorization. Categorized as an illness, ADHD shows evidence of having such features as genetic predispositions and dysfunctions of the mind or brain. So, human agency is after all involved: it is involved in the categorizing or classification of conditions in the light of which the features those conditions have may change.

In addition to the two assumptions criticized by the strong objection to the likeness argument, at the very end of the last chapter a third more fundamental assumption was mentioned, which the likeness argument must make. The likeness argument asks whether or not conditions such as schizophrenia are illnesses or not: this is how it answers the radical question Szasz raises. If these conditions prove to be illnesses, the likeness argument says, this will show that mental illness exists.

But perhaps radical questions such as does mental illness exist and is schizophrenia an illness and so on are asked in a rather different way from the way the likeness argument presumes. Perhaps, rather than being questions about whether there is anything that meets the conditions for being a mental illness, these are questions about the idea or concept of mental illness. Perhaps to ask does mental illness exist is not to ask: Is there anything out there that is a mental illness? but rather to ask: Does the idea of mental illness make sense? Perhaps when we ask is ADHD an illness, we are actually asking whether the very idea of ADHD makes any sense. The question may be: Is it even possible to apply the notion of illness (enshrined in ADHD) to the behaviours that

DSM-IV (for example) describes (American Psychiatric Association, 1994, pp. 83–5)? And perhaps, when the sceptic says that mental illness does not exist, what is being suggested is that the very notion or category mental illness makes no sense. And if the sceptic argues that there are no such illnesses as schizophrenia, ADHD, or alcoholism, what is actually being argued is that it makes no sense to apply the notion of illness to the sorts of things ideas such as schizophrenia, ADHD, and alcoholism are applied to.

This chapter will start to ask about this way of taking the radical question, and about a sceptical response to the question and the possible reasons for giving it. The question at issue will be: Does the sceptic have good reasons for arguing that the very idea of mental illness is unintelligible, or that it is nonsense to try to apply a notion such as ADHD to, say, the behaviours it is usually applied to?

To answer these questions, we need first to understand what sort of thing mental illness as an idea is. Once we understand that, we can begin to ask how it is to be questioned. I shall suggest that mental illness is a classificatory concept. I will argue that this means that whether it makes any sense as a notion—whether it is intelligible—cannot be settled by any form of empirical investigation. Rather, we will need to look at the component parts of the idea (mental and illness) and assess how well they fit together conceptually. Similarly, the questions whether schizophrenia, alcoholism, or ADHD are illnesses are also questions about coherence. In these cases it is whether the notion of illness coheres with the way in which we identify and describe the behaviours that are said to characterize these conditions.

I will start by asking what classificatory concepts are, and making some observations about them.

Classificatory concepts

When we assert or deny that something exists, we can mean more than one thing. We can mean that this thing has no instances, or we can mean that it can have no instances. To deny that the earth's second moon exists (for example) is to deny that there are any instances of this thing, or, simply, to deny that earth has a second moon. To deny that there are planets orbiting distant stars is to deny the existence of those bodies. These are both examples of denying that something exists by denying that it has any instances.

The likeness argument asks whether there are any instances of mental illness. It sets off from a generic account of illness (e.g. dysfunction, action failure) or from some specific agreed paradigmatic illness (e.g. hypertension or more broadly physical illness) and asks whether putative mental illnesses (e.g. schizophrenia or alcoholism) are of the same kind. Those who use the likeness argument ask, in Boorse's words, what a theory of mental health (and hence mental illness) should be. They do not doubt that such a theory is possible, that is to say they do not doubt the category exists. Those who deny the existence of mental illness on the basis of the likeness argument would be arguing that there are no instances of it—for example, by arguing that schizophrenia or bipolar disorder are not really illnesses.

However, we can also deny that something *could* have any instances. That is we can say it's impossible to classify any object in that way, because we deny the existence of the kind itself, of the whole category.

We have constant recourse in our ordinary conversation, in our academic discussions, and in our imaginings to classifications and categories. For example, *planet* is clearly a category of things. The concept planet refers to a kind or class of thing. That is to say it plays the part of helping to distinguish things into types or categories. Planets are distinct from moons, asteroids, and stars. Jupiter is a planet, but Ganymede (a moon of Jupiter) is not, nor are any of the asteroids orbiting the sun in the asteroid belt planets, and nor is the sun itself. Having the category planet and other categories enable us to distinguish between objects in respect of the kind of thing they are said to be.

These are distinctions that we do not have to make, and have not necessarily always made in the way we presently do. At a time when it was thought that all heavenly objects (except the fixed stars) orbited the earth, so that Saturn, Jupiter, and Mars were thought to act like the Moon, the distinction between moons and planets was not needed. But when it was suggested both that Saturn and the others in fact orbited round the sun, and not round the earth, whereas the Moon orbited the earth, and that Jupiter had heavenly bodies orbiting it, the distinction between planets and moons was made. In English, a trace of ambiguity remains, which may go back to the time when these distinctions were first made: we name the earth's moon the Moon.[1]

If we ask the question do planets exist? the answer seems to be, obviously, yes, they do. However, what evidence do we have that planets exist? Certainly, we have the evidence that particular planets exist, such as Saturn, Mars, and Jupiter. There is some evidence that planets exist in orbit around other suns. But that is not the same as having evidence that planets exist. Saturn's existence is not evidence that there are planets, as Saturn can be a planet only if planets exist. All the evidence that individual examples of the kind planet exist depends on us identifying certain things as planets in the first place. We have to have the category planet already to do this. The question do planets exist is not necessarily the same as a question about whether Saturn (or any other individual planet) exists. Rather, it may be about whether there is any such kind of thing as planets. It may be asking: is there any such class or category?

It is my argument here that mental illness is a classificatory concept, and that the radical question of the existence of mental illness is a question about the concept rather than about the things the concept may be said to refer to.

The role and nature of classificatory concepts

Put aside the question of whether I am right about this for a moment. The nature of the claim becomes clearer when we consider the role and nature of categorical concepts. Two things may be said about these. (1) Categorical or classificatory concepts play an organizing role in our experience of, responses to, understanding and explanation of the world,[2] and (2) are not (ultimately) given to us by the evidence of our senses (though of course we have to learn to use the concept from other people). These two statements amount to saying that the claim that mental illness is a classificatory concept is not an empirical claim, not a claim based upon observations or upon experiment and evidence. Rather, it is a conceptual claim. This will emerge in this and the following subsection on coherence and examples.

When it is said that mental illness plays an organizing role in our experience of the world, I mean that it enables us to make sense of and indeed to have certain experiences. We come across someone who behaves in a way we consider odd, or bizarre, even frightening or perverse, claiming to be pursued by the CIA or that her thoughts are being broadcast over the television. How are we to understand what is going on? To do so, we have various ways of classifying such people. We may regard the person as eccentric, as many did in the case of Salvador Dali. Or we may regard the person as nasty, or evil, as is the case with Hitler and Stalin. Or, we may regard the person as insane, as was the case with nineteenth century poet John Clare and artist Richard Dadd. Eccentric, evil, and insane are ideas that we apply to the behaviours of people we find around us, and by means of which we may begin to make sense of those behaviours. Indeed, for the sake of completeness, I should note that my original descriptive terms 'odd, or bizarre, even frightening or perverse' are themselves classificatory, though they may not be explanatory in the way eccentric, evil, and insane purport to be.

These categories—evil and ill for example—not only play a putatively explanatory role, helping us to understand some of the phenomena we may come across. They also become part of our experience. We will not be able to experience someone as either insane or evil, and not as odd or bizarre, if we lack these categories.

In this sense classificatory concepts make experiences possible. This is a statement that can be taken at two levels. We can consider the role of categories at the specific level, as in the cases just given. Or we can consider it at the most general level, where we would be looking at the role of such concepts with respect to our experience as such.

On the general level, a view has been developed by philosophers[3] that, if we did not have a range of concepts with which to organize our experience, it would be difficult to know just what our experience would be like. Indeed, it might be hard to say if we would have any experience at all without the use of some set of classifications. Among the ways in which we organize our experience which I have mentioned as we have gone along have been: groups of objects, such as musical instruments, birds, and planets; different kinds of trees, such as house-building trees and date palms; I have referred to various categories of disease such as pneumonia and cancer. I have also mentioned more abstract categories such as likeness and difference, function and dysfunction; and so on. Any developed language offers a rich variety of such classifications.

However, nothing I am arguing depends on holding the general thesis that only if we have classifications can we have experience. On the more particular level, where our concerns chiefly lie, what is held is that some specific experiences are made possible only by specific categories. Peter Winch gives an example in *The Idea of a Social Science* of how classificatory concepts make particular experiences possible.

> [S]omeone with no understanding of the problems and procedures of nuclear physics would gain nothing from being present at an experiment like the Cockcroft–Walton bombardment of lithium by hydrogen; indeed even the description of what he saw in those terms would be unintelligible to him, since the term 'bombardment' does not carry the sense in the context of the nuclear physicists' activities that it carries elsewhere. Winch (1990, p. 84)

In this case, whatever someone without the relevant concepts would experience were he to see scientists carrying out the 'bombardment' of lithium by hydrogen, or would understand by this description, it would not be what physicists who have the concepts in question experience in observing or understand in describing the Cockcroft–Walton experiment. Of course, he would experience (understand) something. Perhaps he would think it was an experiment, perhaps even an experiment in physics. These are categories or concepts one may well have even though one is not a physicist oneself. By means of these concepts he could make some sense of what he was seeing, distinguishing it from a religious ceremony or a sports event, for example. Winch's point is that the physicist's experience would be inaccessible and its description unintelligible to someone without the necessary conceptual foundations.

How the acquisition of concepts may play a part in influencing our experience can be illustrated with an example used by Ludwig Fleck, the Polish philosopher of science. He invites us to look at a black and white image, without telling us what it is an image of. In this state of ignorance he offers us a number of descriptions of details of the image, when seen from close to: 'From the black background the picture of a gray, wrinkled surface stands out. Some places look like rough folds, others like densely arranged warts, one place reminds us of the waves of a muddy liquid, others of clouds of smoke (perhaps because the picture in this border place is out of focus).' (Fleck, 1986, pp. 129–30).

These descriptions are possible in ignorance of the nature of the image given the range of familiar concepts Fleck has available to him, just as a lay description of the Cockcroft–Walton experiment can be given. Having made such detailed descriptions, Fleck offers us a number of possible accounts of what the picture as a whole is actually of. He suggests that it might be the magnified skin of a toad, or a culture of the penicillin fungus (p. 130). In fact, as he goes on to reveal, it is neither of these, but a photograph of a cirro-cumulus cloud (*ibid.*). With this information about the kind of thing the picture represents, Fleck invites us to admit that looking from afar,[4] we now 'see immediately the enormous depth of the sky, and a large fluffy cloud whose variable structure, while unimportant in the details of the limited places, in its entirety reminds us of a sheep's fur', which previously had been obscure to us (*ibid.*). Merely given the image to look at, we can apply various concepts to its interpretation. When we look at the picture not knowing what it is, it does not determine what concepts should be applied to its interpretation, or what descriptions should be made of its detailed features. When we know what the picture is of or correctly apply the concept cirro-cumulus cloud we come to recognize a set of detailed features appropriate to the whole of which they are details. Again, Fleck's point is that what we know influences what we see. The experience of looking at the picture in ignorance of what it is a picture of is transformed by finding out that it is a picture of a cloud.

These examples are of specific images (cirro-cumulus clouds) or events (the Cockcroft–Walton experiment), and it is with the specific and particular that our concerns lie. Mental illness plays a categorizing role offering the possibility of experiencing people exhibiting certain phenomena as being ill. In this it is parallel to the instances described by Winch and Fleck.

More importantly for my purposes, it is the existence of the concept of mental illness (or the application of the concept illness), which makes possible the likenesses between examples of human conditions such as schizophrenia or alcoholism or ADHD and others such as pneumonia, or essential hypertension. As the strong view of the mistake in likeness arguments suggests, to think that the features of schizophrenia give us the idea that it belongs to the category of illness (is a mental illness) is to get things the wrong way round. Schizophrenia acquires the features of illness (such as dysfunction) in being categorized as one, just as Fleck's mysterious image acquires the features of a cloud by being categorized that way.

If mental illness is a category or classification of things, organizing and making possible certain experiences and explanations, then it follows that the category cannot be acquired or derived from experience. And again, depending on the generality of one's analysis, two routes are available to show why the category mental illness is not derived from experience. If one holds the very general thesis that categories organize experience or make it possible then one can very quickly arrive at this conclusion. If it is the categories that make experience possible, then it is impossible to acquire any category from experience, including of course mental illness. Any experience we have will already be categorized, in which case the categories have already been applied and hence must already have been acquired from some other source prior to the point at which we experienced anything. Of course, even holding this general thesis, it would be accepted that each of us acquires at least some of the concepts within which we organize our experience. We do this in the course of learning and growing up. The general thesis is not that we are born with all of them. And, what we learn we learn in experiencing, for example when we are children from observing and listening to our parents and responding to them. Nevertheless, the general thesis would hold that learning how to use a category and having the experience the category enables us to have at the very least come together.

However, my thesis is not the more general one, but the more modest particular one. I do not want to say that no categories are derived solely from experience, rather, the notion of mental illness is not derived in this way. In the case of mental illness, the concept goes into our experiences of people. The experiences and the concept come together; they are a package, if you like, and you cannot have one without the other. We have somehow to learn the concept by coming into contact with it in our childhood or later, and this inevitably means we come into contact with it in experience. However, once we have acquired the concept the role it plays is to make certain experiences possible, experiences that were not possible before we had the concept.

One can offer some tangential support for the idea that having the category is necessary to being able to experience or explain things in its terms. If one looks into history, certain individuals who might now be regarded as mentally ill were clearly not so regarded in their own time. Joan of Arc heard voices and believed she was called by God to lead France to victory over the invading English. People at the time were divided over whether to think of her as an instrument of God (a Saint) or of the Devil (a witch). No one however argued she was ill. We would now have this as a possibility, even if we did not use it (see also Reznek, 1991, pp. 23–4, and Drury, 1996, pp. 123–4). Western culture has acquired the concept of mental illness in the meantime.

If we look at contemporarily contentious diagnoses, such as ADHD, we find something similar. How are we to understand the behaviours of some adults (such as Carl Elliott's friend Grady) who zone out in meetings or seem unable to advance in their jobs? At one time, explanations would have to have been in terms of personal failings, psychological problems, or perhaps in terms of the boredom of the meetings or the nature of the jobs. But the expansion of the ADHD category to adults (see Conrad and Potter, 2000) provides a further explanation—in medical terms.

It is the nature of classificatory concepts such as mental illness (and more specific diagnoses such as ADHD) to make possible certain experiences, responses, understandings, and explanations. It can also be seen as the foundation of any notion that the things referred to as schizophrenia, alcoholism, or ADHD have features that belong to illness. Indeed, in the case of certain of these features (genetic causality for example), the application of the concept is part and parcel of the presence of these features. And of course, the existence of the concept is necessary to its application. If the concept does not exist, then it cannot be applied.

Coherence and examples

The quotation at the start of this part of the book is from Wittgenstein, and is to the effect that in order to know what is being looked for it is useful to know how the looking is being done. I suggested that this can be transmuted into the idea that how one goes about answering a question tells one something about how one understands the question. If the question *does mental illness exist* is a question about the intelligibility of the category (or concept) of mental illness, how would one go about answering it? I want to suggest in this subsection that the answer cannot be discovered by means of investigating whether there are any examples of mental illnesses: it is by no means an empirical question. We cannot answer it by reference to the contingencies of the world. This is because, in a very radical sense, looking for examples of mental illnesses in order to establish whether mental illness as a concept is intelligible, or coherent would be a waste of time; neither failing to find nor finding an example would establish the case.

On the one hand, if we fail to find an example, it will not show the concept is incoherent. For example, it has been suggested that the Earth has two natural moons or satellites: the Moon, and one other, a much smaller object. From time to time astronomers have gone searching for this second Earth moon, but without success. (There are many other similar examples of objects believed to exist in space, for various reasons, but which have never been found: for example Vulcan, a planet supposed to orbit the sun closer even than Mercury, and on.) However, though a second Earth moon has never been found, this does not mean that the idea of a second much smaller moon orbiting the Earth is incoherent. There might indeed have been such an object, though it is believed pretty much certain these days that there is not. There would indeed be little point in searching for this object these days: but this would be because surely if it did exist it would have registered on some instrument by now. The chances that it is there but we have simply missed it are vanishingly small. But it would not be pointless looking for it because an object of that description could not possibly exist.

On the other hand, even finding an example of something is not what shows the concept of that thing is coherent. We will have known before we found the example that we had a coherent concept, for if we had not we could not have been looking for an example of it. We can intelligibly say we are looking for the second Earth moon, and this shows we have a coherent concept. However, we cannot intelligibly say we are looking for an example of an incoherent concept such as: a straight line that is not the shortest distance between two points; a triangle with four sides; an integer that is both odd and even. It is not that history suggests our chances of finding any of these objects is vanishingly small. It is because it is not possible for there to be any of them. They are impossible ideas. Straight lines just are the shortest distance between two points, at any rate in Euclidean geometry; triangles are three-sided figures; and integers are either odd or even, and cannot be both.

In fact, with incoherent ideas like these, it is not strictly speaking a waste of time looking for examples of them. Rather, it is not really possible to *look for* examples of them; the idea of examples of such things is itself confused. An integer that was both odd and even would have to be divisible by two and not divisible by two; but no integer can have both these properties at the same time. Any integer we choose to look at will be either odd or even, and we know that right from the start. We know that in order to collect triangular objects we will have to search for objects with three sides. If we find an object with four sides, we shall say that it is not triangular. There is no logical or conceptual space for a four-sided triangle. Only things for which there is logical or conceptual space can be exemplified, and only things that can be exemplified can be sought for.

If mental illness is an incoherent idea in the way that a four-sided triangle is an incoherent idea, then there will be no examples of it, certainly. But, more important, there *could* be no examples of it, and we would not know how to go about looking for examples.

And if mental illness is an incoherent concept then we will not be able even to ask questions such as: is schizophrenia a mental illness? A parallel instance is the current argument about whether Pluto is really a planet or not. Some astronomers are now inclined to think of Pluto as one of a vast number of non-planetary objects in what is called the Kuyper Belt. This disagreement about what kind of thing Pluto is is possible only in virtue of the existence of concepts such as planet and Kuyper Belt (for a recent survey of this and other related issues see McKinney, nd, pp. 16–19). Similarly, the question is schizophrenia a mental illness relies for its existence upon the concept mental illness.

Further, if the concept mental illness is incoherent, the likeness argument will also be incoherent. The likeness argument starts with a search for putative examples of mental illness preparatory to assessing whether they bear sufficient resemblance to physical illnesses to be called illnesses too. However, one cannot have a putative example of something of which one cannot have an example. And one cannot have an example of anything which is incoherent. In short, nothing which cannot possibly exist can have anything in common with something which either does or could exist.

When it comes to assessing the coherence of concepts or categories, examples are out of the picture. We will have to look at the concepts themselves to find whether they are incoherent or not.

3.2 A coherence argument against mental illness

In this section and in the rest of this chapter I want to investigate a case for saying that mental illness is an incoherent concept. This case is that the notion of illness makes sense in a frame of reference that is distinct from—and excludes—the frame of reference in which the notion of the mental makes sense. (I could replace the phrase *frame of reference* by *standard of description* or *set of descriptive tools*.) One of the things I shall try to do is to suggest what accounts of these two frames of reference might be given. One possible account is that illness falls into a physical frame of reference, while the mental falls into the non-physical. This may suggest that the basis for the incoherence argument is something like Descartes' mind–body dualism. However, it will emerge that it need not be. Another frame of reference for the notion of illness seems to be what we might call the natural while the frame of reference for what is called the mental is plausibly the human-made, i.e. the social, moral, political, and so on. In either case, these two frames of reference are distinct and exclusive, and so do seem to be a good foundation for the incoherence argument. Notwithstanding, as will become apparent, I shall argue that neither dualism is a good enough reason for rejecting the notion of mental illness. None the less, it leaves us with a question how the concept of mental illness could come about. And the answer (to be given over the course of the rest of the book) will be that it comes about by a process of imaginative recategorization: by metaphor.

The incoherence in mental illness

The incoherence in the phrase *four-sided triangle* lies in the fact that using the notions four-sided and triangle together leads to inconsistency. A triangle used in the usual way implies a closed figure with three straight sides; and this is in itself coherent. Four-sided is on its own quite coherent too. It is a term we can use in many descriptions. A square, a rhombus, and my office are all four-sided. The incoherence lies in the combination of the two ideas. Neither mental nor illness appear to be incoherent in themselves. So, the task for someone who thinks that mental illness is an incoherent concept is to show that the mix of ideas within the concept is impossible.

Those who have plausibly gone some, or all of the way down this route include Thomas Szasz, Karl Jaspers, and Kurt Schneider (in what follows I will focus largely on Szasz). Jaspers and Schneider seem to imply that the frame of reference that is applicable to illness is the physical. Healy reports that 'Both Jaspers and Schneider argued that the normal use of the word illness implied that something physical must be disordered' (Healy, 1990, p. 61). Jaspers, referring to the diagnostic schema of mental illnesses in the early twentieth century, notes the belief that the major psychoses (which were taken to be epilepsy, schizophrenia, and manic depressive disease) would prove to have 'a somatic base'. They would then be categorized with somatic illnesses that caused psychic disturbances (such as infections and General Paralysis; Jaspers, 1997, pp. 605ff). Healy concludes: '[I]f the neuroses are not illnesses and as the psychoses are mainly physical rather than mental illnesses (even if psychologically precipitated) are there any mental illnesses? A conclusion that the Jasperian revolution points towards is that there are no mental illnesses; that mental illness is a logical impossibility' (Healy, 1990, p. 61).

Szasz also I think tries to capture something of this logical or conceptual impossibility in his arguments. He says that the notion of illness goes with the physical. The organs of the body can be sick (he uses the words illness, disease, sickness, and their various derivatives synonymously). 'The liver' he says 'can be sick; the heart can be sick' and sick here means 'that there is something biologically amiss with a part of the body' (Miller and Szasz, 1983, p. 272). Heart and liver are organs or systems of the body; they are physical. When we speak of illness we always mean physical illness. So there is no room for an illness of anything that could be called or qualified by the concept mental. And conversely, whatever descriptive resources can be applied to the mental, descriptions in terms of illness are not among them.

Brain diseases

At this point a question arises: why not accept that mental illness simply means physical illness but of a particular organ, namely the brain. On this account, it would be describable in terms of the physical matter of the brain, or in terms of the physical as opposed to the mental frame of reference. Szasz holds that the brain is an organ and can be diseased (cf. Miller and Szasz, 1983, p. 272). Early nineteenth century psychiatrists (alienists) seem to have thought the same, claiming that madness must be a somatic (physical) disease. Jaspers seems to have believed that the psychoses (schizophrenia and manic depression) were brain diseases, comparing them with epilepsy (see Healy, 1990, pp. 61, 70). Moreover, those who clearly believe in mental illness tend to think of it as being brain based. As we saw earlier, Anton (2001) defines alcoholics' craving as a state of the brain. Sir George Still (often claimed as an early observer of ADHD) explains certain rather trying behaviours he observed in some children in terms of brain disease (see Still, 1902). And modern medical histories of ADHD all assume that a species of brain abnormality is at the bottom of it (cf. Barkley, 1997; Accardo and Blondis, 2000).

The objector to the incoherence argument says that this suggests that mental illness is not an incoherent idea at all. The distinct characteristic of mental illnesses is their mental (psychic) symptoms—that is to say the beliefs, behaviours, attitudes, and so on in terms of which they are usually identified. So, for example, when the symptoms of the brain diseases are beliefs about one self such as 'I am Napoleon' or 'I am being pursued by communists' we tend to refer to mental illnesses. But, the claim against the incoherence argument goes, we do not mean that anything mental is ill—we mean the brain is ill.

However, it can be argued that this does not show that the notion of mental illness is coherent after all: on the contrary. Szasz, for example, argues that where such beliefs are so-called symptoms of illness they 'would be considered mental symptoms *only* if the observer believed that the patient was *not*

Napoleon or that he was *not* being persecuted by Communists' (Szasz, 1982, p. 21; Szasz's italics). The judgement that someone is not what he says he is 'entails . . . a covert comparison or matching of the patient's ideas, concepts, or beliefs with those of the observer and the society in which they live' (*ibid.*). This, says Szasz, shows that these so called symptoms of mental illness are of a quite different kind from those found in physical illness.

Szasz says: 'The notion of mental symptom is . . . inextricably tied to the *social* (including *ethical*) *context* in which it is made in much the same way as the notion of bodily symptom is tied to an *anatomical* and *genetic context . . .*' (*ibid.*; see also Brown, 1985, p. 554).

In support of Szasz's point here, we may contrast the sort of judgements entailed in the case of pain (a bodily symptom) with those in the case of beliefs. The former do not involve judgements of a normative kind, says Szasz. Pain in illness is tied to the anatomical and genetic in the sense that it is to these contexts that we look to explain the pain and understand its implications. In contrast the question, is this person Napoleon as he believes himself to be, implies a different sort of approach.

It might be responded that Szasz's point is clearly contradicted by the possibility that a report of pain is a lie. However, this line of argument turns out to support rather than undermine Szasz's distinction. The argument would be that when we receive a report of pain, we make a normative judgement about whether or not the person is making it up before we refer it to the bodily context for explanation. This, it might be claimed, is similar to making judgements about the patient's beliefs about who he or she is. However, while tempting at first, this response in fact supports and identifies the difference to which Szasz refers, that is to say the difference between what he would say are genuinely symptoms and what are in fact something else. When we doubt that Mr Smith is in pain we doubt he is being honest with us: that judgement does involve a moral aspect. That would be equivalent to doubting, in a parallel case, that Mr Jones really did think he was Napoleon (perhaps he's just saying he does to fool us or to get out of a nasty spot). But if we accept that Mr Smith is indeed in pain, our next question seems to be what causes it. This is does not imply a further normative judgement, and this is when we start to think of it as a symptom. But, Szasz argues, we do go on to make a further judgement about Mr Jones claim to be Napoleon, which is that this is a bizarre claim, and one he must be wrong about.

If one has no reason to think that someone who believes something odd (I am Napoleon) is displaying a symptom of anything, one has no justification for trying to correct any physical abnormality that might be associated with it. Whereas pain may indicate that something is wrong with the body, so-called mental symptoms do not indicate that there is anything wrong with the brain. In short, insofar as mental illnesses necessarily involve such beliefs or other things mental, there is no justification for thinking of them or any supposed physical basis of them in medical terms. That is the wrong kind of judgement to apply to them, the wrong kind of framework of thinking or set of descriptive resources.

Underlying Szasz's worries here are the implications of ignoring this fundamental difference of approach. He is concerned that the slip from beliefs and attitudes to symptoms lifts a bar between medical and moral or more broadly social judgements. This is why, I think, Szasz refers to psychiatry as being the 'medicalisation of morality' (Miller and Szasz, 1983, pp. 285, 286; see also Healy, 1990, p. 1) and one reason why he so strenuously opposes the idea of mental illness. His counter-argument that mental illness is incoherent suggests that this bar cannot be lifted conceptually speaking. Whatever we may say, the incoherence argument goes, beliefs and attitudes are not symptoms of illnesses.

The incoherence argument, then, says it makes no sense to try and force together the notions of illness or sick and mental or mind. Nothing from the physical world of diseases can be caught by the mental world of the mind. Simply 'The mind . . . cannot be sick' (Miller and Szasz, 1983, pp. 272–3). Mental illness is conceptually, or logically, impossible, like a four-sided triangle. If we use the concepts mental and illness, mind and sick in the way we usually use them, there is no logical space for mental illness. Mental illness is an incoherent concept.

This is certainly a strong statement of the ideas of sceptics such as Szasz. And I'd like to raise a couple of questions about it. The first question is what these ideas are based upon: how can Szasz be so sure that the two frames of reference or sets of descriptive resources are incompatible? Can we find a good basis for this claim? I will start the exploration of this question in two ways. Under the subheading *A first objection to dualism* I will consider the suggestion that Szasz's incoherence argument rests upon a general idea that mind and body are two quite different sorts of things. This general idea is that of Cartesian or substance dualism. This, it can be argued, would be a problematic basis to rest the incoherence argument upon, as it is often accused of being incoherent itself. I will argue, however, that this is not the only basis Szasz could choose, and is in fact not the one he does choose. However, arising from this objection will be a second, that Szasz has failed to account for the possibility of mental dysfunction. This will be considered under the subheading *The idea of mental dysfunction.* If it is accepted that someone arguing that mental illness is incoherent has to make allowances for the notion of mental dysfunctioning, this also means that any dualism of the mental and the physical (whether substance dualism or some other sort) may be the wrong dualism to rely upon.

A first objection to dualism

The first potential objection is that the incoherence argument is relying on a division between standards of description—or frames of reference or tools of description as I called them earlier—which is not sustainable. The division in question is the division between mind and body that is seen, for example, in Cartesian (or substance) dualism. The objection to the incoherence argument goes that it is the Cartesian dualism that the incoherence argument is said to be relying on which should be rejected, not the idea of mental illness.

This is not the place to go into the details of Cartesian mind–body dualism, even supposing I was able to do so. Some very general claims about it will have to suffice. As just mentioned, applied to humans, the classical dualist holds that they are entirely made out of two kinds of things or substances (see Descartes, 1981a,b, particularly Principle LIII, p. 240). One substance is called matter and is a physical substance, and the other substance is called mind and is a mental substance. For the Cartesian dualist, these two substances are utterly different from one another: as different as a thought from a house, a memory from a hose, or an attitude from a horse. One could certainly argue on the basis of such a belief towards the idea that mental illness is an incoherent idea. Given the complete contrast between the two substances, if illness is a state of the physical substance, it cannot also be a state of mental substance.

The objection the incoherence argument is facing is that if this is the basis of the argument that mental illness is incoherent, it is a flawed basis, and the argument is therefore likewise flawed. It could be argued that mind–body dualism is not flawed, but such an argument would not be easy to make, might well fail, and would in any case be misleading. My response on behalf of the incoherence argument is to point out that incoherence arguments against the notion of mental illness do not necessarily rest on a Cartesian dualist basis, and so objections to such a basis will not necessarily undermine the incoherence argument.

Szasz, for example, is not a Cartesian dualist.[5] He does not have to worry about any flaws in substance dualism, at least not in the way a Cartesian dualist has to. A Cartesian dualist thinks mind is a substance, but Szasz thinks that mind is a part of our way of talking. It is a sort of short-hand, a collective term for a whole range of things that we sometimes want to contrast with body. He says: 'the mind is an abstract noun that lacks a concrete referent' (Miller and Szasz, 1983, pp. 272–3). The mind is not a substance but a feature of the language. So, while Szasz does indeed claim that the mind is not an organ of any sort, he does not further claim that mind is made of mental substance, or indeed, made of anything. And because Szasz thinks mind is a collective term, or abstract noun, for things we want to contrast with the body, he can conclude that it cannot be diseased or ill, 'Since the mind is not a part of the body, is not an organ—since the mind is an abstract noun that lacks a concrete referent—it cannot be sick' (Miller and Szasz, 1983, pp. 272–3). In short, a coherence argument against mental illness does not have to rest upon an implausible Cartesian dualism (and thankfully I do not have to establish whether or not Cartesian dualism is flawed).

However, even though Szasz is not a substance dualist, he is a dualist of a certain sort: that is say he believes that the descriptive resources that apply to the body—and in particular the descriptive resources offered by illness terms—do not apply to anything other than the bodily organs. When it comes to describing whatever collection of things mind refers us too, another set or sets of descriptive resources is/are needed, or so Szasz argues.

The idea of mental dysfunction

An objection to Szasz's dualism is still available, however. It is that, though he is not a substance dualist—he does not think mind is a substance—he still uses a contrast between the body (the physical) and some collection of things which is broadly speaking mental. But, surely there is something which is mental which has a fair claim to being capable of being ill, namely anything that could be described as a mental function.

When we earlier looked at descriptions of conditions such as schizophrenia (in Chapter 2 on the likeness argument) we noticed claims that this condition represents a dysfunction. Frith describes schizophrenia as a failure of the self-awareness function. In a subsequent chapter, we will see that Barkley describes ADHD as a breakdown of the inhibitory and other functions. Self-awareness and inhibition can be construed as mental functions—functions of the mind, if you like. Admittedly, the relation hypothesized between such mental functions and the brain is usually very close (as is indeed the case with both Frith and Barkley). But neither altogether abandons the mental realm (see Chapter 7 for an analysis of the role of this in Barkley's theories of ADHD). Their ideas receive support in philosophical accounts of illness. Philosophers Boorse and Wakefield construe disease/disorder wholly or partly in terms of mental dysfunction (cf. Boorse, 1982; Wakefield, 1992a,b). Not everyone agrees (cf. Fulford, 1989), but the existence of mental functions seems to have some support.

Sceptics have not been slow to notice that the idea of mental functions is important in many defences of mental illness. Szasz claims (and objects to the fact) that the notion of illness expanded in the nineteenth century with the idea of functional diseases (cf. Szasz, 1974a, pp. 12–13, 36). One can see why Szasz might want to object, given his scepticism. If the notion of dysfunction is rightly applied in the case of physical illness it does not seem all that much of a problem to extend it to the mental. Moreover, it is not clear that Szasz's form of dualism (between physical things such as organs of the body and linguistic things such as the mind) gets round this. Mental functions might be the kind of thing we use the collective noun mind to refer to, but they are not like claims such as 'I'm Napoleon' or 'My thoughts are being broadcast on the TV'. Accounts in terms of dysfunction seem to be plausible descriptions to give if, for example, the short-term memory is not working (as in Alzheimer's disease), or the mind's self-monitoring as awry (as in Frith's account of schizophrenia).

A sceptic (even if not Szasz) can, however, accept the idea of mental functions, such as those to be found in Frith's account of schizophrenia, and yet continue to hold that the notion of mental illness is incoherent. It is true to say, I think, that the traditional mental/physical distinction does not seem to provide any basis for the incoherence argument in this case. But the difference between what might be regarded as natural on the one hand and what might be regarded as human made (or social) on the other does seem to. For example, this difference can be applied in the case of schizophrenia, as described in the previous chapter. Frith's claims that schizophrenia is an illness go with his notion that it is a dysfunction of the self-monitoring function of the mind, while Boorse's account might go with his notion that schizophrenia is a failure of the reality checking function of the mind. These we might think of as failures of the natural or biologically given functions of the mind. However, if we take the alternative, non-illness account of schizophrenia, which focuses on our beliefs about or conceptualization of the self, or the care or carelessness with which we check the truth of what we say, this fits in well with the idea of socially produced norms and practices.

So, if we want to accept that there are mental functions and dysfunctions, a dualism of natural (on the one hand) and the social (on the other) seems a better basis of any incoherence argument than is any form of mind–body distinction. Moreover, the natural–social dualism is based on a form of dualism that has a basis in the literature. This basis is the natural–social dualism of those whom Latour defines as moderns (cf. Latour, 1993, p. 10ff). Latour argues that modernism (or the 'modern critical stance' p. 11) has practised (or at least believes that it has practised) purification. By purification, Latour means the division of the natural (non-human) world from the social (human) world. Latour bases some of his ideas on a book by Shapin and Schaffer (1985) which is an account of the seventeenth controversy over the possibility of a vacuum between Boyle and Hobbes. Latour notes that Shapin and Schaffer—writing in a modernist vein—seem to believe that the rift between nature and society is discovered and developed in the course of this controversy. Boyle, they argue, creates the concepts (the tools of description) that we apply to nature ('experiment', 'fact', 'evidence', 'colleagues'; p. 25), whereas Hobbes creates the concepts we apply to power or, more broadly, the social and political ('representation', 'sovereign', 'contract', 'property', 'citizens'; pp. 24–5).

The modernist's apparent purification of the world into the non-human and the human (or social) would underlie the claim that mental illness is an incoherent notion in this way: By offering two descriptive frameworks, one for each of the two notions (mental and illness), which are quite distinct from one another and cannot be interchanged. Moreover, it seems natural (as it were) to place the notion of illness in with other supposedly natural things (natural categories, natural forces or whatever). Moreover, if illness is a natural thing (discoverable by experiment, the subject of facts and evidence) then it is not to any degree made by people (p. 30). To claim that illness is in any sense made by people—that it is something to do with society or the political, with our beliefs, attitudes, and behaviours—is, on this account, to contaminate or to confuse the notion of illness.

The incoherence account can then recruit this form of dualism to its cause while allowing for the idea of mental dysfunctions. They may be described in illness terms. But, when it comes to the phenomena of those things we usually class as mental illnesses, a sceptical line can still be taken. When someone claims that he or she is Napoleon, or chooses to drink to excess despite the harm, or is not inspired by school lessons or board meetings, we still have no justification for calling these symptoms or thinking that they are evidence of illnesses. We may not agree that the person claiming to be Napoleon is who he says he is, or make the moral judgement that people ought not to drink to excess or ought to overcome feelings of boredom to attend in class or at work, but that is all to do with various beliefs, attitudes, and values. Judgements such as these are human, socially made things, not to be found in nature.

A second objection to dualism

But, even as I have been introducing Latour's idea, and using it to support a sceptical position I have been setting out the foundations of an objection to it. Just as substance dualism is a wrongheaded picture of the relations of mind and body, this objection states, so too purification of things into purely natural and purely human is a wrongheaded picture of relations of the natural and social. Latour argues that this purification is an invention of the modernists. He says the actual picture is much more dynamic and mixed. He refers to the idea of hybrids, illustrating what he means by these with the ozone hole. He starts by noting how stories in newspapers such as those about this hole run together 'science, technology and society' (1993, p. 3). Hybrids 'would link in one continuous chain the chemistry of the upper atmosphere, scientific and industrial strategies, the preoccupations of heads of state, the anxieties of ecologists' (p. 11).

A similar picture of mental illness can easily be produced: the killing of a man by another with schizophrenia may have politicians under attack for failing to fund the psychiatric services or psychiatrists defending their decision to release someone into the community, while other scientists debate the nature of the problem we call schizophrenia perhaps arguing about the most effective medical response. The objection would say that it would be dogmatic to hold that the man with schizophrenia could not be ill because illness has the natural and not by any means the social as its frame of reference. The objection holds that these frames of reference are themselves artificial.

It may well be, then, that even if we understand the basis of the incoherence argument as being a dualism of the natural and the social, we will still not have found a good foundation for it. We'll see, none the less, that both mind–body and natural–social dualism have been employed by those who have argued over the reality of mental illness. For example, in Chapter 6 we shall see how doctors sought to use the idea of mind–body (or perhaps soul-soma) dualism to establish their claims that mental illness was actually within their (physical) ambit. And in Chapter 7, we shall see how social constructionist arguments about ADHD rely on the idea that what is made by humans cannot be illness.

So far I have been quite defensive about the incoherence argument: I now want to look more positively at some of the ideas upon which it rests. The fundamental and extremely plausible notion it seems to express is that concepts have boundaries.

3.3 The incoherence argument considered

The idea of appropriate descriptions

It seems obviously right that we cannot apply a concept to simply anything we like. Some things are and some things are not planets, colours, triangles, numbers, and straight lines. We make a mistake if we call the moon a planet, because the concept planet refers to things that orbit stars, and moons orbit planets. The boundary of a concept goes with the idea that we cannot apply it wherever we feel like it. Conversely, it means that in most cases we cannot describe things just as we like. Given we have a concept and some idea of what it means, it will be appropriate in only some particular cases to describe things in terms of this concept.

In fact, the whole idea of classification seems to rely upon constraints of these kinds. If there is too much in the way of overlapping and extension of concepts we seem to be in danger of losing them altogether. This problem can be called the underdetermination of concepts and can be found in discussions such as that of Bellaimey (1990), which we mentioned earlier. Bellaimey, whose discussion focuses on the family resemblance approach to concepts, argues that, as everything is like everything else in some respect, likenesses between things cannot be the sole basis of categorization. If they were, every particular thing would eventually turn out to be categorizable as the same kind as every other particular thing. Everything would turn out to be a member of every category of thing, and under these circumstances the notion of a category loses all its grip. Some kind of restriction is needed.

In Chapter 2 we rejected the idea that this restraint on the application of disease and other central medical terms is created by the features that things are supposed to have. None the less we can recognize that this idea was trying to get at something important. That important thing is the relationship between the concept under which something falls and the descriptions we give of the thing.

We sense in very many areas that some kinds of descriptions go with some kinds of thing but not with others. And this is the point behind the objection to the idea of mental illness that we have been discussing. To use a terminology that we shall employ again: there is an internal relation between descriptions of this kind and being an illness. For the sceptic, descriptions of illness must be disconnected from beliefs, attitudes, and so on. These are moral and social things, and they should be described in social and political terms. This means, for the sceptic, that they cannot be connected with illness descriptions. They are connected with social, political, and moral value judgements; that is what they are internally related to.

So, we know our concepts have some form of limit of application. However, to deny that we can apply illness to the mental is applying this idea in a place where we may not be used to seeing it applied.

Is the purely conceptual objection to mental illness convincing?

But the language is not always so tidy as the idea that concepts have boundaries makes it appear. We can disagree about what should fall under a concept (see Beardsmore, 1992): is bull-fighting a sport, or not? Is schizophrenia an illness or not? And how do we decide? The fuzziness or untidiness of concepts is to be found all over, and so too the lack of clear guidelines on how to decide questions of this sort. The likeness argument tries unsuccessfully to supply these guidelines in the case of mental illness. And it goes wrong just because things in this particular area cannot be cleaned up in the way it thinks they can. We cannot find features of schizophrenia that tell us it is a mental illness.

However, ideas that seem in many ways to be quite different do turn out to have exactly those sorts of connections it may seem they should not have. For example, the mental and the physical, which Szasz wants to keep apart. The mind is often spoken of as if it were a sort of container or a location. We say we will bear some idea *in mind*; we talk of bringing some memory *back to* mind. Someone who feels sad (which is presumably a state of mind) is often said to feel *blue*. Some ideas are described as more *weighty* than others. And, of course, we talk of mental illness, despite Szasz's opinion that we should not or cannot do so. Nor is this Humpty Dumpty talk. There is nothing extraordinary about this: words that apply to physical things seem quite frequently and ordinarily to be used to describe mental things (cf. Empson, 1951, p. 331; Lakoff and Johnson, 1980 *passim*).

True, no one makes the mistake of looking up in the air for a high mood, or down to the ground for a low one. That is to say we do not confuse high feelings with high things. It can be argued that these examples of linguistic flexibility are merely ways of speaking. It's a fact about words that they have this flexibility. However, it can be said that it's not a fact about how the things described in this way really are. A description can be literal and straightforward, but it can also be fanciful.

Usually we do not confuse our more fanciful descriptions with our more mundane or prosaic ones. However, people who are medically qualified do diagnose people with schizophrenia, give them drugs, and treat them to all appearances as if they were patients, in places called hospitals which are built and funded from the health care budget. This appears not to be merely a way of speaking, not purely a verbal matter. We may not look up for a high mood; but we may well look for a mentally ill person in the psychiatric wing of the local hospital.

Moreover, the linguistic side of psychiatric talk seems perfectly natural, as if it had a proper home among the concepts within which we understand the world around us. The concept mental illness, despite protests that there can be no such idea, is found and widely used within the language, as Szasz (1973, p. 48) notes. There does not seem to be anything in the grammar or semantics of the language preventing us using it. In contrast a phrase such as 'I see a voice' seems to break some rule. Four-sided triangle seems patently absurd in a way mental illness does not strike us as being. Mental illness is as familiar a usage as in mind and out of mind. Furthermore, it appears to coexist quite easily with the continued use of terms of a social, ethical, political, and religious kind; the two frames of reference continue in existence alongside the treatment of those said to be schizophrenics, alcoholics, and adults with ADHD. Most importantly, the term mental illness seems capable of *use*. It is, as we pointed out at the start, woven into much of our social organizations and institutions, in our judicial and constitutional arrangements. It is difficult to see how anything supposedly absurd as a four-sided triangle could play such a part.

In what sense, then, could mental illness be without sense?

What's wrong with mental illness

I want to take up Szasz's response: he thinks we need to recognize that what is wrong with the concept of mental illness is that it involves metaphor (see also Sarbin, 1969, p. 19, cited in Boorse, 1982, p. 32).

> Szasz's (1971) main concern has been to extend his insistence that minds can be sick only in a metaphorical sense (like economies) in order to show how the notion of mental illness has acted as a smokescreen in modern times, hiding subjugation and ill-treatment of non-conformists by the State.
>
> Pilgrim (1992, p. 215; the reference is presumably to *The Manufacture of Madness*)

Minds are sick metaphorically. They are sick in the same way as economies are sick; or that an argument is cast-iron; or that a memory is distant. These are familiar English phrases. And they are all metaphorical. They all involve a combination of ideas that other uses of these words should prevent. An economy may well be said to be sick. We may even say that a good economist can *diagnose* the problem and *prescribe* a *remedy*: but we do not actually call in a doctor. Everyone knows that economies are not biological organisms or people; so no one makes the mistake of co-opting a Hospital Consultant to the Treasury; and there is no branch of medicine along the corridor from Neurology and Gynaecology and Obstetrics, called Economy. In short, no one is at all fazed by talk of sick economies; nor do they think there is some special meaning of the word sick that applies to economies; they know that sick economy is not to be taken literally. And this is, as Pilgrim says, how Szasz thinks of mental illness.

Indeed in Szasz's mind, if I may so put it, this is not only how it is but it is absolutely obvious that this is how it is. The following bald example is intended to demonstrate just this blinding obviousness.

> By screwdriver we ordinarily mean a tool used by carpenters; we also give this name to a drink made of orange juice and vodka. Clearly, saying that the drink is a metaphoric screwdriver is not saying that it is some other kind of screwdriver; it is saying that it is not a screwdriver at all. Similarly, if I say that mental illness is a metaphorical illness, I am not saying that it is some other kind of illness; I am saying that it is not an illness at all. Szasz (1987, pp. 150–1)

Against Szasz's example, we might say that he is confusing a homonym with a metaphor. However, that aside, Szasz's point is clear enough: You cannot treat, cure, diagnose, or in any way conceive as medical a mental illness; and parallel to this point, you cannot screw a screw into a piece of wood with a vodka and orange. Metaphorical illnesses are no more illnesses than metaphorical screwdrivers are screwdrivers.

Szasz's description of mental illness as metaphorical is not an additional argument for his position that mental illness is incoherent. The idea that mental illness is metaphorical illness and that mental illness is an incoherent concept come together in Szasz's account. Neither one can claim to be a reason for holding the other. Nevertheless, there is something to be garnered from Szasz's notion that mental illness is a metaphor. And what that is will appear more clearly when we investigate what a metaphor is.

Conclusions

Leaving behind the likeness argument this chapter has considered another way of raising and answering questions about the existence of mental illness. Perhaps the question is about the idea or notion of mental illness. I suggested that mental illness represents a category in terms of which we may seek to organize and understand the world, rather than a category that the world gives us. But perhaps this supposed category involves a mix of other ideas that simply do not hang together. Perhaps the category cannot really exist. I have wanted to offer some mild support to this thought. At any rate, I have sought to suggest that it does not rest upon what might be regarded as a problematic basis in substance dualism. I have pointed out two other forms of dualism that it might also rest upon. These were Szasz's form of mind–body dualism and Latour's modernist dualism of nature and society.

What such dualisms may seem to help explain is something significant. And that is the fact that ideas such as mental and illness but also any others you might care to mention have boundaries. They cannot be applied to just anything: they have to have limits. So this leaves open the possibility that mental illness is indeed an incoherent notion. The two notions of which it is constituted may have boundaries such that further ideas connected to mental and further ideas connected to illness are quite distinct from one another.

This idea of limits is in turn related to an idea that Thomas Szasz uses—the idea of metaphor. Metaphor is a combination of ideas that seems to be deliberately incongruent or incoherent. Szasz says mental illness is just such a combination. As will emerge in the next part of the book, I think Szasz has hold of some element of the truth here. But the element of the truth he has hold of does not ultimately support the idea that mental illness is an incoherent idea: rather, it serves to explain the nature of its existence. Mental illness is indeed a metaphor.

Endnotes

1 Though we also use the term satellite instead of moon. Another example similar to moon and The Moon is the term galaxy. Astronomers refer to the galaxy in which we are located as The Galaxy (cf. Arendt, 2004).

2 A notion commonly found in literary theory; cf. Richards (1936) (cited in Empson, 1951, p. 331), and Abrams (1953, p. 31).

3 I have in mind Kant's transcendental categories and space and time (1961). Hacking (1983, chapter 7) draws attention to different ways in which a transcendental account may be cashed out, contrasting Kant's transcendental idealism with Putnam's transcendental nominalism.

4 Fleck is interested in the contrast between looking at the details of the image, and looking from afar at the image as a whole. We get the general impression that the room is somehow different: we then look for the particular piece of furniture that has been moved or changed. We do not infer or deduce the difference because we see that a piece of furniture has been moved or changed (see Fleck, 1986, p. 130). A related idea may be that of *gestalt*, the sense we get of the whole of something, which in turn depends upon the various wholes we are capable of being aware of. See also Wittgenstein's discussion of the duck–rabbit (1992, pp. 194ff).

5 Boorse agrees (see 1982, p. 32). Reznek disagrees (see 1991, p. 147). He points out that Szasz believes that the mind is not a bodily part (p. 72) and that beliefs we have reasons for cannot be caused (p. 74). He speaks as if these conclusions could be reached only by someone who holds substance dualism. Szasz's view of the mind can perhaps be inferred from his reference to Gilbert Ryle, and in particular to the notion of a category mistake, in his interview with Jonathan Miller (1983, p. 272; cf. Ryle, 1973, particularly chapter 1).

Part 2

Metaphor

4 Metaphor

4.1 Introduction

This second part of the book has two principal tasks. The first, which will be taken up in this chapter, is to explore what might be meant by metaphor. The aim will be to show that and how metaphor may be a means of reclassifying or recategorizing things. This idea of metaphor will be contrasted with the claim that metaphor is a deceptive use of language for social or political purposes. I will instead advance the idea that it is a way of making the world. Mental illness, as a metaphor, represents the world made in a certain way. It does not represent a socially convenient fiction about how the world really is.

The larger point is that some of what the world is is down to how humans make it. We make it in the sense that we apply categories and classifications to it, which in particular cases make possible our experiences of the world. However, our classification or categorization of the world is not fixed. We can shift these categories, breaking down their boundaries, or using them to bring a particular set of concepts to bear in an area where previously another set of concepts were to be found. The sign in language of this kind of breaking of boundaries, and consequent remaking of the world, is the metaphor. The metaphor of mental illness is a case in point.

The second principal task of the two chapters in this part of the book is to bring together the idea that metaphor is a way of remaking the world with the arguments of the weak and strong views, and particularly the latter. The strong view says we do not assess the kind of thing alcoholism, ADHD, or schizophrenia are upon the basis of their features or likenesses; rather the features of such things appear in the light of the kind of thing we think they are. Metaphor marks an alteration in our views about the kind of things schizophrenia and other such conditions are. When we change our views about this, we change the features these conditions can be said to have. I will consider two examples that illustrate the work of metaphor. Both of these will come from physical medicine, rather than psychiatry.

This will lay the groundwork for the third and last part of the book, where some of the ideas developed here will be applied in the area of mental illness.

4.2 Metaphor as fiction

In the first part of the book we saw that one sceptical approach to mental illness is to say that it is an incoherent idea. Szasz, for example, makes this claim when he says that mental illness is a metaphor. For Szasz, a metaphor entails a straightforward and simple falsity, or lie. His account is not original, but reflects a view to be found throughout the history of thought about metaphor. It has its source near the beginning of that history. Szasz takes his lead from Aristotle whose definition is he says 'still as good as any': 'Metaphor consists in giving a thing a name that belongs to something else' (Szasz, 1987, p. 137; Aristotle, 1941, p. 1479).

We might think of the wrong naming in the notion of mental illness in various ways. Most obviously it would consist in giving the name illness to something such as schizophrenia, which is not an illness. It might lie in using the term ADHD to name a particular claimed pattern of inattentive, hyperactive, and impulsive behaviours. Or it might be said that the metaphor would lie in using the adjective mental to describe the noun illness. Those who hold that mental illness is an incoherent notion, among them Szasz, would say that illness cannot have a mental character. Szasz might cash this out by arguing that illness relates only to physical things such as the organs of the body. But we have pointed out that an alternative and perhaps a better way of describing the border between illness and the mental is in terms of the natural and the social. By illness we mean something naturally made. You cannot have an illness of anything that is constructed or produced by humans—illnesses are always connected to things created by nature. As beliefs and values are human creations, so the incoherence argument might go, they cannot be ill. And as so-called mental illnesses involve such things as values and beliefs, they cannot be examples of illness. Such things, as Szasz might put it, could be called illnesses only metaphorically.

However, though Aristotle's definition of metaphor is, in Szasz's eyes, a good start, it does not go far enough. Giving something the wrong name may be an aesthetic ploy, a mistake, a misunderstanding, or a joke. However, none of these describes what Szasz thinks about metaphor. More than merely wrong naming, Szasz says metaphor involves deception as it 'involves the pretence that something is the case when it is not' an idea he claims to derive not from Aristotle but from Turbayne (Szasz, 1987, p. 138; Turbayne, 1970). The deceptions involved in the notion of mental illness are the pretence that things such as schizophrenia are illnesses, when they are in fact not illnesses; or the pretence that some illnesses are mental in character when they cannot be. According to Szasz, Turbayne's is clearly a different point from Aristotle's, and does not follow from it.

The fact that metaphor for Szasz involves wrong naming and pretence does not entirely invalidate its use even for him. However, it can be used only in certain circumstances and for certain purposes. Szasz gives (and approves) C.S. Lewis's view that 'We must use metaphors. The feelings and imagination need that support. The great thing... is to keep the intellect free from them: to remember that they are metaphors' (Szasz, 1987, p. 139; quoting Lewis, 1981, p. 145). Lewis and Szasz's approach has a predecessor in Hobbes (cf. *Leviathan*,

1975, I, viii, pp. 136–7) as Szasz notices (cf. Szasz, 1987, pp. 138–9). All three hold that, though metaphor has its place in the emotions and in the imagination, it must be segregated from the intellect.

For Szasz, in sum, mental illness, in being a metaphor, entails a falsity, or lie. It takes the form of wrongly naming something. However, in matters of reason and intellect these falsities must be exposed for what they are. The implication of the idea of mental illness is that we can talk about, and treat, thoughts, beliefs, attitudes, ideas, and the people who have them, as if they were subject to disease. In fact, Szasz argues, they cannot be, and it is straightforwardly wrong and pernicious to claim they are or could be (cf. Szasz, 1973, p. 48; 1979, pp. 34–5 (cited in Reznek, 1991, p. 77); Boyle, 1990, p. 179). The metaphorical character of the notion of mental illness spreads to all the medical terminology applied to the mentally ill (see Szasz, 1987, p. 140). But no matter how far it may spread, the real purpose of the idea of mental illness is hidden by the metaphor. He argues that that purpose is to enable the control of certain awkward members of society.

My approach in what follows will be to consider the notion of metaphor and ask whether a usage that is, as Szasz claims, wrong in some sense might not be deceptive so much as creative and imaginative.

4.3 Categorical metaphor

I shall not attempt to define metaphor; or what we must mean if we say that mental illness is a metaphor. I shall want to accept that metaphor can mean something very close to what Szasz says it means, though not that it must involve deception. It can, as Szasz says, refer to bringing two things under one name, though I shall want to talk about bringing two things under one concept. This bringing under a concept is reflected in the verbal forms that metaphors take. On the surface of it, wrong naming is still correct. I shall call the form of metaphor I am interested in categorical metaphor (another possible choice is classificatory metaphor).

A standard example of a categorical metaphor is 'John is a wolf' where John is wrongly named, or brought under (categorized under) the wrong concept, wolf (cf. Black, 1954–5). Because I am interested in the categorization of schizophrenia and other so-called mental illnesses, I shall be particularly interested in statements that, like 'John is a wolf', take the form '*x* is a *y*'. Our examples will be 'schizophrenia is an illness' or 'ADHD is an illness'; or, more broadly, 'mental illness is an illness' or 'madness/insanity is an illness'.

Szasz's chosen metaphor, mental illness, does not take this verbal '*x* is a *y*' form. The metaphor lies in the application of an unexpected adjective. This is a form day-to-day English language revels in: a weighty idea, a cast-iron plan, a distant memory. So we shall need also to be interested in metaphors of the form 'a *z y*'. A good literary example is 'a green thought' (Marvell, 1972, p. 101).

However, we can unpack mental illness so that it reads 'a mental condition which is an illness' to give it a more obviously categorical feel, which is in turn very close to 'mental illness is an illness' or 'madness is an illness'.

When it comes to phrases such as 'schizophrenia is an illness' or 'ADHD is an illness' we need to unpack things slightly differently. Obviously, in one sense, it is simply true that ADHD is an illness—it is by definition, as ADHD arises from a medical context and takes a medical form. To see the metaphor in these phrases one would need to remember that terms such as schizophrenia and ADHD are here being used as shorthand to refer to a collection of behaviours. For example, ADHD might be taken to refer to the pattern of behaviours described in DSM-IV (American Psychiatric Association, 1994). What is metaphorical is the application of the idea of illness implicit in ADHD, schizophrenia, or alcoholism, for example, to such described patterns of behaviour. We should not confuse the two uses of the words. In fact, 'ADHD is ADHD' could in theory be a metaphor.

In order to say something more about categorical metaphor and about its relation to our concepts, and in particular to our concept of mental illness, I will use a series of contrasts. Metaphor in general is very often and rightly contrasted with other usages of language. In the sections that follow four contrasts will be drawn. And in the course of drawing each contrast an attached contesting idea of what is going on in the use of terms such as mental illness will be introduced. In each case the contesting claim is that something other than metaphor is going on (or, alternatively that metaphor means something other than what I am claiming it means). And in each case I will reject this contesting claim in favour of the idea that the notion of metaphor, construed as a categorization, is the right idea of what is going on when we use the term mental illness.

1. The first contrast with metaphor can be called metaphorical sense, but I shall consider at the same time an idea I take to be related, namely secondary sense. The idea that contests with the thought that mental illness is a categorical or classificatory metaphor in the case of metaphorical or secondary sense, is the idea that illness does not have its usual meaning in the metaphor mental illness. This account holds that the metaphor would not involve categorization of certain behavioural patterns as illnesses in the ordinary understanding of that term. My response is to say metaphor involves the existing meaning of words and not the development of a new meaning. The illness in mental illness is the ordinary meaning of that term.

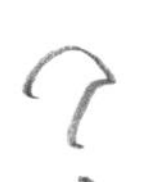

2. The second contrast with metaphor is simile. The idea that contests with the idea that mental illness is a categorical metaphor in this contrast is that metaphors are simply similes (overt comparisons) in a punchy or arresting verbal form (which arises from their being covert comparisons). I shall respond that we need to accept that simile and metaphor may refer to quite different ideas. A simile does not involve the recategorization of things. A metaphor can do—a categorical metaphor does—and the metaphor of mental illness is an example of this.

3. The third contrast is to the wide range of duties a word may ordinarily have in the language, but that do not amount to metaphor. The idea that contests with the claim that mental illness is a categorical metaphor in this contrast is that the word illness has far wider duties than has been allowed for. I shall respond that a categorical metaphor is not an example of such extended duties, and that there isn't a good argument that illness does refer as a part of its usual duties to mental illness.
4. The fourth contrast with metaphor is dead metaphor. The idea that contests with a claim that mental illness is a categorical metaphor in this third contrast is that mental illness was a metaphor but has since developed a sense of its own, which is a metaphor only historically. A dead metaphor is one that has developed a place in the ordinary language, and has lost the impact that a challenge to our usual categories may have. I shall argue simply enough that this is not the case with mental illness.

All four contrasts will prove useful in identifying the use of metaphor I wish to develop in this part of the book.

Metaphorical and secondary sense

In Chapter 2, I mentioned that Richard Gipps argues that the likeness argument actually serves to remind us of something we tacitly already know—that such things as schizophrenia are illnesses. If Gipps is right then my claim that mental illness or schizophrenia is an illness are metaphors would be false. They would involve a categorization, but there would be nothing metaphorical about these phrases if they simply express what we already know or think we know.

However, Gipps adds an interesting further point to his claim that we tacitly know that schizophrenia is an illness, which is that the word illness in this case does not take its ordinary meaning (the meaning it presumably takes in the case of physical illness or in references to pneumonia and so forth). Rather it has a special sense: what Gipps (2003) calls a secondary sense.

Secondary sense is an idea that has been discussed by Wittgenstein (1992) and by Cora Diamond (1991). Wittgenstein focuses on examples of uses of words that to most speakers of a language would appear quite odd, for example, the use of the word fat to describe one of the days of the week. Diamond's focus is on some moral terms such as good. In both cases, it is claimed that in the secondary sense of a term something is named that the speaker experiences (the fatness of Wednesday for example). Furthermore, it is claimed that the speaker is not really able to find an alternative word—some other way of describing what they experiencce, unless, that is, it is an alternative word (such as corpulent) for fat. And yet the meaning of fat in relation to Wednesday is not the primary sense of the term.

Perhaps, in what appears to be a categorical metaphor, we find the use of a word such as illness in a secondary sense. Translated into the case of 'man is a wolf' the argument would be that the sense of the word wolf (or perhaps man) in this case is a special one. In mental illness, perhaps the word illness is really the only one that will do, but all the same, it does not have the same implications or extensions as the word illness in its primary sense has.

There is some reason to think that some commentators on metaphor think that in metaphor words change their senses, and take on a metaphorical sense: and this idea is one of the main targets of Donald Davidson's essay on metaphor (1984). (*Metaphorical sense* is also used by Charlton, 1975, to refer to the meaning in a dead metaphor: see below.) Whether this amounts to saying they have a secondary sense is a further question. But we do not need to pursue this question, because for my purposes the issue is somewhat the same in either case. In both cases—metaphorical and secondary sense—the idea that metaphor represents categorizing something such as a pattern of behaviours, beliefs and attitudes into an illness category (or even the idea that metaphor is a wrong naming) seems to be lost. There is no shift into the illness category, because in neither metaphorical nor secondary sense does illness take its ordinary meaning. Rather it takes a meaning that is applicable and appropriate to the mental.

I think Davidson is correct to contend that metaphor does not involve a new sense of its words. Take the metaphor 'a green thought'. If we suppose that this involves a special meaning of green or of thought we are in danger of missing the oddness or challenge that metaphor can represent. If green, for example, has some special meaning in the way fat is supposed to when applied to Wednesdays, we might appear to be restricting the understanding of metaphor to those for whom these uses seem merely descriptive of their experience. If on the other hand we suppose that Marvell had some special metaphorical meaning of green in mind, we appear to be consigning ourselves to a guessing game about what it might have been. I do not think either will do.

There are perhaps special reasons for thinking that the illness in mental illness or mental illnesses has some special sense. Svensson, for example, contrasts what he calls the 'fundamentalist' and the 'metaphorist' approach (see p. 72), and Radden notes a similar contrast (1985, pp. 17–18). Svensson's argument is that mental illness should not be assumed to have the usual meaning of the term illness (which is the meaning that applies in physical illness). This, he suggests, is because it should not be understood or treated in the way that physical illness is understood and treated. Svensson wants, in this way, to reform our approach to mental illness. The desire to reform our approach to mental illnesses—perhaps to encourage a move away from narrow biological approaches, as Antony Clare calls them—is certainly a strong motivation in many of those who are critical of psychiatric approaches.

The problem for Gipps is to say what justification he has for thinking that illness in mental illness or mental illnesses is being used in anything other than its ordinary sense. The kind of explanation we see being given within psychiatry is clearly on a par with other medical explanation: it is causal, often brain based, or sometimes related to functioning. It might be argued that these terms are also being used in secondary or metaphorical senses; however, this seems as much to presuppose as to support the claim that illness is being used this way.

Metaphor, simile, and likeness

Earlier I said that metaphors are assertions such as '*x* is *y*'. They imply recategorization, as when we say 'John is a wolf' or 'madness is an illness'. However, it is sometimes thought that this is a misunderstanding of metaphor. It is sometimes thought that metaphor is essentially a form of comparison. It draws our attention to likenesses we had never thought about before. This is said to be the real purpose of the assertions in question. These claims are all wrong, but there is something important in the idea of comparison that needs to be connected to metaphor: metaphors may create the possibility of comparison.

The linguistic figure that is overtly comparative is the simile. The simile uses the terms like or as. Hence, in the stock example of discussions on these matters, John is a wolf is the metaphor and John is like a wolf is the simile. The simile refers to whatever things John and wolves have in common. But if the metaphor is essentially comparative in nature, then it is not different in essence from the simile: similes are just up-front about it. John is a wolf on this view is just another less explicit way of saying John is like a wolf. Perhaps it is a verbally more striking way of saying this, and hence has aesthetic or poetic merit. But it is not a way of meaning anything different.

Tirrell discusses the idea that 'metaphor is essentially comparative' (Tirrell, 1991, p. 358). She contrasts two possible ways of taking this idea. In her terms, one is to take it reductively and the other to take it non-reductively. Reductive similes focus on the characteristics or features two things share. The reductive simile account turns metaphor into a way of referring to features of likeness between things. Tirrell points out that reductive simile accounts of metaphor are usually rejected. If, she says, a writer can be shown to have the idea that metaphor is really reductive simile by another name, then that is seen as equivalent to showing that he or she has missed the point of metaphor. Black rejects Davidson's account in part on these grounds (see Black, 1980, p. 189). Tirrell herself rejects both Black and Davidson because she thinks in the final analysis they both hold that metaphors are really reductive similes. Tirrell rightly, in my view, argues that metaphor and reductive simile are not the same thing. Metaphor is not another word for comparison of that kind.

The reductive simile account will not do, Tirrell argues, because clearly John is like a wolf is not the same in meaning as John is a wolf. The word like, in its reductive sense, is not otiose. There are many things to which it may be supposed to refer in the case of a person and wolves (e.g. both being mammals, both being social animals). We may extend this analysis to the associated features of John and wolves: for instance to their (supposed) treachery. (This is how Black (1954–55) cashes out his notion of metaphor.) The word 'like' used in a reductive way implies reference to such features of wolves and men as these. Unless we assume that John is a wolf is simply a shorthand for John is like a wolf, we must admit that there is clearly a difference between the meanings of the two phrases. In adding the word like in this reductive sense, something is lost as well as gained. What is gained is the specification of comparison among the features and perhaps associations of things. What is lost is the notion of categorization. As we have already noted on a number of occasions, two things can be like one another without being of the same kind: but one thing cannot be another without being of the same kind.

This leaves Tirrell's notion of non-reductive simile to be explained. Tirrell explains what the word like used non-reductively adds to phrases such as John is a wolf by describing the notion of figurative comparison. When Romeo says of Juliet 'she is the sun', he is making a comparison. However, it is not a literal comparison. It does not rest upon literally shared features. Romeo is not attempting to point out that Juliet, like the sun, has hidden interior processes taking place within her (even though she does, of course). He is, rather, referring to a range of other features of the sun and Juliet that they share figuratively. Both are warm, both lighten Romeo's day, both are his source of life, and so on.

These are figurative likenesses; and for figurative here read metaphorical. The sun is warm, so is Juliet; it is warm in temperature, she is warm in the sense of having warm feelings towards Romeo; the sun warms Romeo in the way it warms the air and oceans, Juliet warms his heart by being in love with him. And so on. Taken altogether out of context, and just to illustrate, we could construe an earlier example 'green thought' as a figurative comparison by noting that both green and thought can be bright. However, the word bright is being used metaphorically in the case of the thought. A bright thought is metaphorically luminous. A weighty thought is metaphorically weighty. And so with warm and light; the sun is warm in temperature, and luminous; Juliet is warm towards Romeo in loving him, and brightens or lightens his day.

Tirrell has an important insight here. To put her point in other terms, the word 'like' is no less capable of being used metaphorically than is any other word. Hence, if we come across the claim that two things are like one another, we have yet to find out whether they are literally alike, or metaphorically—as Tirrell would put it, figuratively—alike. To say metaphor is simile is not necessarily to be reductive. The use of the word 'like' does not absolutely distinguish the presence of simile from the presence of metaphor. In fact, as Tirrell herself admits, it leaves her with the problem of distinguishing non-reductive or figurative simile from metaphor.

The difference Tirrell is looking for is I think the difference between categorization and comparison. Even figurative comparisons do not involve the actual identification of the things compared. Juliet is figuratively like the sun; but she is not the sun. In contrast, I think phrases such as madness is illness or schizophrenia is an illness do imply categorization. Having said that, comparisons may follow from the assertion of identity. Following the bare assertion that alcoholism is an illness found in a metaphor we may begin to find all sorts of further points of likeness.

Szasz identifies (and, of course, is sceptical about) something of this kind in apologies for psychiatry such as this by Seymour Kety: 'Diabetes mellitus is analogous to Schizophrenia in many ways. Both are symptom clusters ... Each may have many etiologies and show a range of intensity from severe and debilitating to latent or borderline ... The medical model seems to be quite as appropriate for the one as for the other.' (Kety, 1974, p. 962; quoted in Szasz, 1987, p. 150).

Kety's argument is clearly a version of the likeness argument. He claims to have identified a series of analogies between a physical disease (diabetes mellitus) and schizophrenia, from which he concludes that they are equally explicable on the medical model. The analogies Kety notices include the ideas that both are symptom clusters, both have aetiologies, both are represented in a range of intensities from 'severe and debilitating to latent or borderline'. Anything, Kety seems to think, which has these features will be explicable on the medical model.

On closer inspection, however, Kety's argument is altogether unconvincing, as likeness arguments typically are. To describe schizophrenia as a cluster of *symptoms* is to assume that it is explicable on the medical model before he starts. The same goes for the notion of aetiology. As for the less obviously medical terminology, such as severe, nothing at all follows from such analogies, if they exist. Frosts and looks may vary in severity too, but the medical model is not thereby applied to them. Kety's claim that schizophrenia and diabetes mellitus are analogous and so can fall under the medical model depends on seeing them under a medical model description in the first place.

But if a metaphor is involved, then the likenesses that appear may turn out to be figurative: that is to say they may appear to be extensions of the identity to be found originally in the metaphor. For Szasz, the extended metaphor (myth, or model) of mental illness goes beyond the use of the word illness. It extends to the use of words such as symptom and aetiology, and on to diagnose, treat, and so on. However, according to Szasz, no matter how far the metaphor is extended by the use of further and further medical notions based upon it and reiterating it, not one ounce of strength is added thereby to the contention that it is not a metaphor. Schizophrenia and diabetes mellitus are as much symptom clusters as Juliet and the sun are the light of Romeo's life. Likewise, I think the notion of the metaphorical would extend for Szasz to the notion of genetic causation and mental dysfunction. He would argue that the mind does not literally dysfunction in schizophrenia, for example. If it dysfunctions, it does so figuratively.

Szasz fears that once one has one metaphor, one can expand it through whole lexicons of related words, building nominal bridges between concepts.

But, he would warn, the kind of bridging which words can do should not be mistaken for how things actually are. Things that can be teamed up in metaphors are not thereby really to be teamed up in our understanding or knowledge. We need to be constantly aware of what he would call an incoherence in such statements as Juliet is the light of my life and schizophrenia is a symptom cluster. This incoherence is all very well in the first case, Szasz might say, where we have art. It is not all very well in the second where we are reputed to have science. Tirrell's reminder that comparisons may be figurative appears to be grist to Szasz's mill.

However, we do not have to follow Szasz all the way to his conclusion. Think once again of the strong objection to the likeness argument. This accepts that there may be a pattern of likenesses between physical and mental illnesses. But the strong objection also holds that some of these likenesses may appear because of how we think of the human conditions in question. I have used Tirrell's analysis to arrive at the suggestion that if the original assignment of kind is metaphorical then a series of metaphorical likenesses and continuities may appear. The original metaphor makes possible a range of descriptions in which likenesses appear. The likenesses Kety identifies can be seen in this way: they represent descriptions made possible by the metaphor. And they appear in rather the same light under the strong view: they represent possible likenesses created by the assignment of schizophrenia to the kind illness. The idea that genes play a causal role in alcoholism can be viewed as a metaphorical extension of this kind; the idea that schizophrenia or ADHD are dysfunctions can be seen in the same way.

This is, of course, just what makes Szasz so distrustful of them. However, if we do not accept Szasz's fundamental idea that a metaphor must represent a verbal deception about how things really are, we can review also how we think of the likenesses created by metaphors.

Words with related duties

We turn now to the third contrast with metaphor. This contrast is between metaphor and words that turn out to have a sometimes surprising range of duties. The contrast is made by Champlin (1989), who is also directly interested in our question about the nature and existence of mental illness, and in Szasz's argument that mental illness is a metaphor. He disagrees. Szasz has gone wrong, Champlin suggests, because, though he understands correctly what a metaphor is, he misapplies it in the case of mental illness.

To illustrate his argument, Champlin invites us to inspect a parallel case. He invites us to think of the word breathing as used in three instances: the breathing of a person; the breathing of a fish; and the breathing of a newly opened bottle of wine before it is drunk. Champlin believes one of these three is metaphorical breathing: the breathing of the wine. With the other two uses, we have a demonstration of the variety of duties a word can have (p. 28). Champlin thinks that the use of the term illness displays an analogous variety of duties, and when combined with mental does not amount to a metaphor. Perhaps he would say that if illness is applied to economies it is metaphorical; but it is not metaphorical when applied to schizophrenia or alcoholism.

Nevertheless, as Champlin admits, Szasz is right to point out that there are clear differences between physical and mental illness. 'Compare' says Champlin 'our talk of someone's being mentally ill and physically ill with our readiness to speak of both men and fish as "breathing".... Am I watching the same process?' Trouble starts when we notice that whereas we know what to say when asked "What do humans breathe?", namely, "Air", the fish I can see breathing through its gills under water does not seem to be breathing either air or water.' (Champlin, 1989, p. 26).

We cannot carry over what appears a central characteristic of breathing—breathing something—from humans to fish. Yet we still want to say a fish breathes. What follows? Champlin reviews what he calls the obvious temptation. This is to say that 'If we and the fish both breathe, and there is something which we breathe, then there *must* be something which the fish breathe' (pp. 26–7). This is the sort of temptation that underlies the likeness argument. The likeness argument starts from the idea that if we call two things by the same name (breathing, illness) then the characteristics of the one will be shared by the other (and indeed explain why we call them by the same name). But if we call two things by the same name and they turn out not to share essential characteristics, then we have a mistaken naming or a metaphor.

Champlin reviews the temptation to say that if one breathes one must breathe something, but resists it. There is nothing fish breathe, and this is a logical discontinuity between fish breathing and human breathing. Fish do indeed breathe, but they do not breathe anything. Analogously, he says, a patient who has had surgery and a soldier shot in battle both have wounds. However, the soldier has been wounded whereas, in most cases, the patient has not. Not all wounds are the results of woundings (p. 27); not all breathing is the breathing of something. However, these logical discontinuities (as Champlin calls them) do not add up to fish breathing being metaphorical breathing (or surgical wounds being metaphorical wounds). Rather: '[b]reathing is a more multi-faceted thing than we have bargained for; our language is, as a matter of fact, full of this sort of thing where one word doubles up to perform subtly different, but related, duties' (p. 27).

These sometimes wide differences of duty do not imply metaphor. Provided the word can be shown to have this duty, metaphor is absent. Breathing has duties with respect both to fish and humans. Hence, despite the differences between fish and human breathing, it is not a metaphorical usage.

Analogously, to take up Champlin's main case, illness, if it shows some logical continuities with physical illness, will not be metaphorical when applied to mental illness. It will be a word with a duty we did not quite expect it to have, but it will be one of its duties and not a supererogatory metaphor.

Szasz does not agree, and the question arises as to why not. Champlin puts Szasz's position like this:

> [Szasz] is saying that so-called mental illness and physical illness are completely different kinds of things linked only by metaphor. The strength of Szasz's position lies in the fact that it is possible to produce a list of striking, fundamental differences between physical and mental illness, which creates the impression that the gulf between them is too great to be bridged except in name only (p. 25).

This is a good characterization of Szasz's view of metaphor. Champlin implicitly holds it himself. Metaphor involves two things between which a gulf of difference lies such that it can be bridged only in the language (cf. Lakoff and Johnston, 1980, p. 3). Champlin also shares Szasz's worries about the role of merely linguistic moves in shaping the world. Like Szasz he believes we should not fall into the idea that names determine concepts. They both hold that we cannot meaningfully call just anything illness, and calling something an illness does not make it into an illness. Where Champlin and Szasz disagree is in the application of the notion of metaphor. For Szasz, the gulf between pneumonia and schizophrenia is one which is too great for one name, illness, rightly to apply to both; in one case it must be a wrong naming. We may give to schizophrenia a name (illness) which belongs to pneumonia; but a name does not make a genuine bridge.

Champlin's response to Szasz is to show that there are continuities as well as discontinuities between mental and physical illness. Despite the fact that it is possible to produce a list of striking differences between mental illnesses on the one hand and physical illnesses on the other, Champlin advances a number of points of continuity between mental illness and physical illness. The gulf is not so great as it at first appeared, and can be bridged in more than name. Szasz is wrong to conclude from the logical discontinuities he identifies that mental illness is metaphorical illness. There are after all logical continuities, though we have to look in the right place to find them (Champlin, 1989, p. 28).

One continuity Champlin mentions rewards further inspection. Champlin points out that it is often thought that the notion of illness is connected to the notion of suffering. We suffer from our illnesses, which is to say, or so it appears, that we suffer in being ill. In physical illness this seems to refer to our experience of pain and other unpleasant sensations and feelings. However, as Champlin points out, some mental illness certainly fails to realize this unpleasantness of sensation. Hypomania and psychopathy hardly involve suffering for the person who is said to have the condition, in the sense that the pain of an ulcer involves suffering for the person who has it: 'Clinical descriptions of hypomania speak of ebulliance, boundless optimism, euphoria and self-confidence; the psychopath is described as showing a cold-blooded disregard for the welfare of others without any signs of unhappiness or remorse.' (p. 27).

However, as in the case of breathing, Champlin warns us against jumping too hastily to the conclusion that what one does not suffer from, in this sense, cannot be an illness. For we are wrongly assuming that 'suffer from' means experiencing suffering. It is as if we thought that suffering from an illness always meant feeling ill (rather as we might have thought that all breathing involves breathing something). But feeling ill and being ill are quite different ideas. Champlin points out that one can feel ill without being ill ('as a result of eating too many little green apples') and one can be ill without feeling ill (as will someone who contracts an infection while in a coma). To be ill is not necessarily to experience suffering. 'Suffer from' can mean being ill and does not necessarily imply suffering. Those with pneumonia and those with hypomania may, in a logically continuous sense, suffer from their illnesses (p. 28), though someone with hypomania may feel quite well. The word illness crosses from one to the other on a bridge provided by the notion of suffering from and the other conceptual continuities Champlin mentions.

Given Champlin's account of metaphor it is not surprising that he views logical continuities as his recourse against Szasz. He thinks (as does Szasz) that he has to find something other than the language to bridge the apparent gap between physical and mental illness. As a matter of fact, I do not think that Champlin's argument works. For one thing, it appears to be a likeness argument. Moreover, there is a counter to it. If we understand 'suffer from' correctly, Champlin says, we see that we can suffer from both hypomania and pneumonia. But why, we might ask, should we think that suffering from hypomania represents a logical continuity with suffering from pneumonia? Champlin relies here on the idea that 'suffer from' is not itself a metaphor in the first case. But it could be one of Tirrell's figurative likenesses. For his belief that it is not a figurative likeness Champlin gives us no good reason. And one can think of good reasons why 'suffer from hypomania' might be a metaphor. We suffer from all sorts of things that are not illnesses: disappointments, unwise marriages, self-doubt. Just because we suffer from all of these we do not see this as any reason to think all are illnesses. We know the fact that we may suffer from all these implies nothing about the sort of logical continuity that might be taken to underlie a likeness of kind. Of course, it may be, as Champlin says of breathing, that 'suffer from' turns out to have a quite unexpected flexibility in its duties. However, it undermines the credibility of Champlin's argument to rely on the unsupported existence of this flexibility in order to establish a consequent case for the flexibility of the word illness.

Champlin's main task is to show that Szasz falsely thinks mental illness is metaphorical illness. It is not clear he succeeds. Notwithstanding, Champlin draws a contrast that is helpful in saying what metaphor can be. That is the contrast with extensions of kind that are supposed to be based upon logical continuities. Metaphor may involve bringing a condition like alcoholism under a certain description or kind irrespective of the likenesses or continuities that appear between it and say pneumonia. But the contrast here should be drawn with care: the existence of likenesses cannot rule out metaphor. Otherwise the account of metaphor seems to be too rigorous. If metaphors are to be found only where there are no continuities at all, it will prevent all sorts of phrases being taken as metaphors that clearly can be taken as metaphors.[1] Even if we choose a poetic metaphor such as 'green thought', it is not impossible to find logical continuities between the ideas brought together, though to do so we may have to go into what things do not have. Neither colours nor thoughts have any physical weight. This is a continuity; but if metaphor applies only where there are no continuities, this is not a metaphor. Yet 'green thought' surely is a metaphor, if anything is. Even more obviously 'John is a wolf' would cease to be a metaphor because there are all sorts of continuities between men and wolves (both are mammals, for example). But again 'John is a wolf' is a metaphor.

Metaphors are not utterly ruled out by logical continuities. If mental illness is a metaphor, there may still be such continuities or likenesses. The point here is that if there are such continuities, they do not play a role in the assignment of kind contained in the metaphor. Having said that, when we extend a category by metaphor then likenesses may appear in virtue of that. The idea that we suffer from both physical and mental illness in a logically continuous sense may be part of what we mean when we say that physical and mental illness are both really illnesses. However, the supposed continuity is not the basis of this view; it comes with it.

This is consistent with the strong view of the mistake in likeness arguments. The strong view accepts that likenesses can be found between alcoholism and pneumonia, schizophrenia and hypertension, mental illness and physical illness. However, it holds that these likenesses come with and do not precede the assignment of kind. The bare assertion that something is of a kind is what is found in the metaphor.

Dead metaphors

Yet one thing must have struck us about the phrase mental illness: Szasz refers to it as a metaphor, but if it is it lacks the fanciful impact of many metaphors. It seems so ordinary. As I mentioned earlier, it lacks the absurdity of a four-sided triangle or 'I see a voice', it does not strike one as overtly poetic. It strikes one as a quite natural use of the language. Similarly, 'You indulge' says William Charlton 'in no flights of poetic fancy if you say that your shares have slumped and your dividends have been cut' (1975, p. 174). For Charlton this absence of fancy is the essence of a dead metaphor. A dead metaphor is found in a sense of a word which has developed alongside its other senses. This sense we can call metaphorical, but it does not now involve a living metaphor.

The distinction between *metaphorical sense* and *living metaphor* can be explained using Charlton's example. Charlton thinks that slumped has a non-metaphorical sense, to 'sink or fall heavily' (*Collins Pocket English*

Dictionary, 1996, p. 467, meaning number 2). This is the sense we use when we talk of someone slumping into a chair. However the word in contemporary usage has another sense '*v* **1** (of prices or demand) decline suddenly' (*ibid.*). This is the metaphorical sense. A metaphorical sense originated (according to Charlton) in a flight of poetic fancy. But it has subsequently become 'a sense in which the semantics of a language permits us to use a word' (Charlton, 1975, p. 174). Indeed, in the dictionary I consulted it is the first listed meaning. But 'a sense in which the semantics of a language permits us to use a word' is precisely what a metaphor is not (this is a point strongly supported by Davidson and Rorty too): 'A living metaphor gets its force from being a use which is not permitted'. Once again we are reminded of the idea that metaphor is a wrong naming, an impermissable application of a word, a recategorization that subverts our current classes and kinds, a usage beyond even its most extended range of duties.

Charlton emphasizes the fact that the senses words have cannot be changed in a living metaphor (1975, p. 173). A living metaphor relies on the fact that the words retain their already existing senses. Davidson (1984, p. 247) makes a similar point (as we have seen when we discussed the idea of metaphorical and secondary sense earlier). Szasz agrees. It is just because illness has not changed or developed its sense in the case of mental illness that mental illness is a metaphor. However a word can change its sense, or develop a new one in parallel with the old, by becoming applied to something it was not formerly applied to. Slump becomes applied to a fall in prices as well as to a heavy fall. Then it comes to mean a sudden fall in prices. But this is to lose the life of the metaphor, not to explain or expound it. Meanings of this kind may develop in our ordinary language for speaking about prices, stocks, and shares, and all sorts of other things. Current English is littered with dead metaphors, such as heart of gold, cast-iron plan, and distant memory. These have come to refer straightforwardly to someone's generosity or kindness, a plan that cannot go wrong, and a memory of an event that took place some considerable time previously. And perhaps mental illness is another example of a dead metaphor.

If so, Szasz would still be right in the sense that he judged that mental illness had something to do with metaphor. But he would be wrong if he thought that the metaphor was still living, that it still represented a flight of poetic fancy. The metaphor mental illness would have transmogrified into a metaphorical sense (as Charlton calls it). It would, to paraphrase Rorty, have 'died off into literalness' (1991, p. 167; 1995, p. 118). This would at least explain why the phrase mental illness seems so ordinary; and why statements such as schizophrenia is an illness seem to some to state the blindingly obvious.

But it does not explain why the notion of mental illness is regarded as an extension of physical illness, which is clearly how it is regarded. The notion of an economic slump is not an extension of the notion of slumping into chairs; there need be no logical continuities here. Rather, after initially being applied metaphorically, i.e. impermissibly, it gradually gained general currency as a quite independent permissible usage. This is not the case with mental illness. Though it has been suggested that it be given its own independent meaning (as we've already noted in the case of Svensson, 1990) it seems fairly clear that it, and specific claimed examples of it, e.g. ADHD are usually regarded as illnesses like any other.

As a metaphor mental illness does not fit altogether comfortably with Charlton's notion of dead metaphor. And the main reason for this lack of fit is to be found in Szasz. He can be seen as seeing the metaphorical in mental illness. He sees the fanciful categorization that it represents. From this we can gather something, significant for both Szasz's purposes and for my own. It suggests why and how the notion of mental illness can be challenged. The critic of a metaphor may emphasize its absurdity, as opposed to its imaginative or visionary quality. (This was precisely Szasz's aim in the example of the word 'screwdriver' which we considered in Chapter 3.) To take up an example from Pasteur's work, though not the one we will be considering later: Dubos (1961) notices how Pasteur's idea that microscopic living creatures (as he imagined yeast to be) could produce chemical change, was taken up by one of his critics (Friederich Wöhler) and used to pour scorn on the idea, simply by means of describing yeast in the terms usually reserved for living creatures, that is simply by using the metaphor.

This kind of *reductio* does not apply to Charlton's example. There would be no point in trying to challenge the metaphorical sense of the word slump. Slump was originally applied to prices in a flight of poetic fancy perhaps, or so Charlton claims. But now the word slump has a new sense in which it applies ordinarily to falling prices and demand. This application is straightforward and, except for the historical facts about how it came about, as literal as any other sense of the word. Little hangs on whether the economic sense of slump really is a metaphorical sense. If it turned out not ever to have been a living metaphor, Charlton would have chosen a bad example, but nothing much hangs on the actual history of the word slump.

It is quite different with phrases such as schizophrenia is an illness and other specific examples of that kind. A very great deal may hang upon their history (a point we shall follow up in more detail when we look at social constructionist approaches to ADHD). If this is a metaphorical sense and represents the historical and continuing use of a living metaphor, then it is a historical fact that these concepts have come to be grouped together in the way they are. And that means we can reassess whether we want to go on in the way history has appeared to determine for us. The dead metaphor can be revived, and things having been categorized once, can be recategorized. Schizophrenia (or ADHD) can cease to be an illness.

Whether Charlton would accept this way of taking his ideas I do not know. Perhaps he would not think that what has come to seem semantically acceptable can be made to seem semantically unacceptable again. But the language does not merely expand by accretion, with all its older parts remaining intact, and all new building work going on on new sites. Wittgenstein's famous image of language as a city, with its old parts a tangle of small streets, and some of its newer parts (such as the symbolism of chemistry) looking like 'new boroughs with straight regular streets and uniform houses' (1992, p. 8), is potentially misleading, and in the same way so is Rorty's coral reef image (1995, p. 118). Whole areas of this city can be razed and rebuilt over the years. We can reject a former practice, and in doing so we reject the language that was part of that practice, perhaps eschewing the kinds of description it allowed, the categories with which it worked. If there was once a part of the city in which witches, witchcraft, and the Inquisition flourished, it is now a memory, long ago demolished, and even partly built over. The sceptic, such as Szasz, would like to demolish the area of town called psychiatry. A sceptic about say schizophrenia or ADHD would like to demolish the streets where these notions are domiciled.

Charlton usefully reminds us of the temporal dimension of the development of language. There is one other element of Charlton's position that I wish to adopt. Charlton views metaphor as originating in a flight of poetic fancy. You may recall, from the previous chapter, C.S. Lewis's claim that metaphor is vital to the imagination. Suppose this is applied to the notion of mental illness. The idea of mental illness appears to be part of the conceptual foundations of psychiatry. It represents the work of categorization from which the descriptions of psychiatry arise. But it may also represent a leap of the imagination. This places poetry, or let us say the poetic or creative imagination, in the very heart of the science.[2]

Conclusions

When a sceptic like Szasz calls mental illness a metaphor he means that the idea is incoherent. Metaphor may be taken to express this scepticism because it can be taken to be a reference to a wrong naming, or, as I have argued, to a categorization of something that seems to be wrong. There are ways of understanding what it might mean to call mental illness a metaphor that could in theory show something rather less sceptical. Metaphors may be said to use words in unusual senses, so that mental illness does not really mean what it seems at first to mean. Or metaphors are sometimes taken to be implicit similes (comparisons without their explicitly comparative words). Or what looks like a metaphor may, on further inspection, turn out to be a word taking on an unusual, but not completely inexplicable duty. Or what is called a metaphor may be without the life that a true (i.e. a living) metaphor has. It is, in this case, just a word with a history that involves metaphor, but that has now 'died off into literalness'.

But I have argued that the meaning of metaphor is none of these. A metaphor is a wrong naming, that is to say, it involves the categorization of one thing as a kind or type of thing it isn't. So, the sceptic such as Szasz is right to claim that it expresses the incoherence that he believes marks out the notion of mental illness.

But he is mistaken if he thinks that just because mental illness is a metaphor, or incoherent because it involves categorizations that are wrong, that this shows that we should abandon the idea of mental illness. Some writers are explicitly or implicitly worried that such arguments as this confuse the work of the imagination with the task of science. But I hold there is something right about making the claim that the creative imagination, call it poetic if you will, lies close to the heart of medical science. Indeed, I shall say that the claim that madness is an illness, and that ADHD is an illness are examples of just such a creative imaginative leap. That is something I shall be considering in more detail in the last part of this book, starting in Chapter 6. In the next chapter, I shall consider two examples as a way of illustrating how the creative imagination may have a place not in psychological medicine, but in physical medicine.

Endnotes

1 Indeed if, as Davidson (1984, p. 257) claims, everything is like everything else, metaphor would be altogether ruled out.

2 For views similar to this, see Davidson (1984, p. 246) 'Metaphor is a legitimate device not only in literature but in science, philosophy and the law; it is effective in praise and abuse, prayer and promotion, description and prescription'; Hesse (1980, p. 111) '...the deductive model of scientific explanation should be modified and supplemented by a view of theoretical explanation as metaphoric redescription of the domain of the explanandum'; MacCormac (1976, pp. 35–7, 72) 'Without metaphor...scientists could not change the meanings of terms and suggest new hypotheses'; Rorty (1991, p. 162) 'Philosophers of science like Mary Hesse have helped us realise that metaphor is essential to scientific progress' (see also Rorty, 1995, and Black, 1954–55).

5 Two metaphors from physical medicine

5.1 Introduction

In the previous chapter I began a discussion of the idea of metaphor. Towards the end it was suggested that metaphor is to be found in the heart of science. In this chapter I will continue this discussion by giving examples of metaphors in science. The examples given come from physical medicine. If metaphor can be shown to be at work in physical medicine it may be easier to accept that is at work in psychiatry.

The reason for wanting to show metaphor at work in physical medicine is the, perhaps understandable, concern that to accept that mental illness is a metaphor is in effect to undermine psychiatry. The way I have understood metaphor gives some apparent grounds for this concern. I have argued that metaphor is a linguistic form in which names are wrongly applied—or so it is often said. For example, names that seem to come from the world of the physical or biological may turn out to be applied to the social or human world. In the previous chapter I suggested that a metaphor can mean simply categorizing a thing—in the imagination—as one kind rather than as another. On this basis, all sorts of comparisons (figurative comparisons) may become possible between things. The behavioural and cognitive phenomena called schizophrenia may become imaginatively a symptom cluster.

Writers such as C.S. Lewis and Thomas Hobbes have warned against what metaphor can do if misapplied. Metaphor is unruly: indeed I have described it in terms of breaking accepted boundaries of concepts. Loughlin, criticizing my claims about the likeness argument, cautions against the kind of scepticism that may follow from embracing the ideas in the strong objection to the likeness argument. He was worried about the idea that the way we look at things determines what sort of thing they are and what features they may be said to have. This is certainly my view: if the strong argument is right, the features of things do come with the kind of thing they are thought to be. And if metaphor is at the bottom of categorizing, then this would surely only add to concerns such as those of Loughlin. In embracing the claim that mental illness is a metaphor, without taking on board the cautions of Hobbes, Lewis, or Szasz, I may seem implicitly to have accepted the consequences of embracing a kind of free-for-all in the way in which things are categorized. There seems in my approach to mental illnesses to be no rational basis for their classification.

However, in this chapter I want to point out that metaphor has a place in medical science outside psychiatry. I shall give two examples in which the role of the human imagination in physical medical science can be seen both on a very large scale and in much smaller scale instances. The large scale example involves the use of the idea that the body is a machine; the smaller scale example involves the use of the notion of vaccination in the nineteenth century. Let me start with this smaller scale example. In this I shall try to show how Pasteur *creates* the notion of vaccination through the use of metaphor.

5.2 Pasteur's chickens

Pasteur and vaccination

Towards the end of the eighteenth century, Scottish physician Edward Jenner observed that people (in the first instance, milk maids) who had had a mild disease called cowpox did not succumb to the much more serious and disfiguring disease smallpox, which was highly contagious among the rest of the population. Having noticed this, he guessed that by deliberately giving people cowpox one could protect them against smallpox. Jenner developed this practice, and it became known as vaccination. The word vaccination itself reflects these bovine connections.[1] Until French scientist Louis Pasteur came on the scene in the later part of the nineteenth century, the term vaccination referred only to this practice established by Jenner.

René Dubos takes up the story:

> Pasteur had begun experiments on chicken cholera in the spring in 1879, but an unexpected difficulty interrupted the work after the summer vacation. The cultures of the chicken cholera bacillus that had been kept in the laboratory during the summer failed to produce disease when inoculated into chickens in early autumn. A new, virulent culture was obtained from a natural outbreak, and it was inoculated into new animals, as well as into the chickens which had resisted the old cultures. The new animals, just brought from the market, succumbed to the infection in the customary length of time, thus showing that the fresh culture was very active. But to everyone's astonishment, and the astonishment of Pasteur himself, almost all the other chickens survived the infection. According to accounts left by one of his collaborators, Pasteur remained silent for a minute, then exclaimed as if he had seen a vision, 'Don't you see that these animals have been *vaccinated*!' Dubos (1961, pp. 113–14, Dubos' italics)

Dubos comments: 'To the modern reader, there is nothing remarkable in the use of the word "vaccination," which has become part of the everyday language. But this was nearly a century ago. Then the word vaccination was used only to refer to the special case of injection of cowpox material for inducing protection against smallpox' (Dubos, 1961, p. 114).

As Dubos says, there is nothing remarkable to our ears in Pasteur's words, but to the ears of Pasteur's contemporaries, there would have seemed something remarkable in what Pasteur said. Dubos draws our attention to the unusual use Pasteur makes of the word vaccination. There is something of the incongruity of metaphor in Pasteur's use of this word; a categorization that seems wrong; a tendentious extension of duty; a wrong naming. Assuming this points to a use of metaphor, what might be going on here? What work is the human imagination doing here?

In using the term vaccinated with this reference, Pasteur is both changing it, and not changing it.

He is changing it in the following sense. Up to that time, it had referred to protection against smallpox by the inoculation of cowpox. Pasteur uses it to refer here to the inoculation against virulent chicken cholera by non-virulent chicken cholera. In doing this he makes the application of the term vaccination to vaccination against smallpox a special case of something that can also refer to inoculation against chicken cholera by the use of chicken cholera.

There is also a sense in which Pasteur does not change the term (for everyone or immediately or, importantly, permanently). For it is the wrongness of the application by the existing criteria that expresses his vision. If it was not wrong, odd, or incongruous, Pasteur's colleagues would not have noticed anything in his words. Pasteur would simply have been using the word vaccination as it was supposed to be used, and nothing unusual would have been expressed in its being used to refer to the survival of some of the chickens. However, according to one of his collaborators, something visionary seemed to have been expressed, and the verbal surprise experienced at the time at the very least marks that.

Remaking vaccination: observation, likeness, and metaphor

The view that Pasteur is using his imagination and misusing the term vaccinate can, however, be challenged. It might be argued that Pasteur was expressing an unusual capacity for observation. He has noticed something, something that could have been seen (and perhaps, no sooner had he said it, was seen) by his colleagues. This is not metaphor, it is a word discovering a new duty; it is not a wrong naming, a nominal bridge, but is based upon a continuity which Pasteur noticed. This allows for an apparently unusual use of the word, without necessarily committing us to the idea that it was a misuse, a metaphor. And it does not suggest the creation of anything, or the use of the imagination, because Pasteur is supposed only to have noticed what was already there.

Moreover, it has good scientific credentials. Scientists typically claim to have seen things which are odd or remarkable. Galileo saw moon-mountains. These, on contemporary beliefs, should not have been there, for it was axiomatic that the moon was a perfect body, not subject to earth-like imperfections (for a brief account see Chalmers, 1990). Galileo's claim that there were mountains on the moon may, then, have sounded very odd, on first hearing, rather like a metaphor. However, the oddness turned out to be in the heavenly bodies. It was, if you like, an observed oddness, not a logical (verbal) one. Galileo did not have to use his imagination; he had simply to look.

Applying this to Pasteur, what might he have observed? The most obvious parallel would appear to be the survival of the chickens. This, like the moon-mountains, was a quite unexpected feature of the observable world. However, this is not what we are trying to account for. It is Pasteur's exclamation that what he and his colleagues were seeing was vaccination, which we want to explain. The Pasteur example is not then merely an example of being surprised at what the world may throw up.

It may instead be suggested that what Pasteur and only Pasteur saw was the connection between the survival of the chickens and their earlier having been given another dose of chicken cholera. However, this will not do either. Undoubtedly Pasteur did recognize that the chickens that survived were the ones that had earlier been inoculated with another strain of chicken cholera. But even if Pasteur had been the only one there to notice that, his ejaculation clearly refers to something more. If which chickens survived was what was at stake, Pasteur could have exclaimed 'Don't you see? It's the chickens we inoculated in the summer that have survived, and not the others!' In exclaiming that they had been vaccinated, Pasteur is doing more than reporting which chickens had survived.

If Pasteur did observe something, then, what else could it have been? The strongest candidate seems to be likenesses between inoculation by weak chicken cholera against chicken cholera and vaccination (as understood by Jenner). The idea is that these likenesses are what were noticed by Pasteur, and that they explain his outburst, and his way of putting things. The verbal usage would have sounded odd because only Pasteur noticed the likenesses. Because initially only he noticed these, only he was able to make the extension of the category of vaccination that follows from seeing the similarities; only he realized that there was a new duty for the word. In short, a likeness argument seems to apply here. Pasteur was not making a leap of imagination; rather, he had noticed something and simply drew the obvious conclusion.

The likenesses in question would presumably be described in terms of the general concept of inoculation by disease against disease of which Jenner's vaccination and the chicken cholera inoculation are both examples. The idea is that Pasteur recognizes that vaccination is not the name of a particular process (the protection of humans against smallpox by the inoculation of cowpox) but is rather the name of something more general. And he comes to this conclusion because he notices that both vaccination with cowpox against smallpox and inoculation with mild chicken cholera that protects against virulent chicken cholera share the features that describe the more general concept of vaccination.

The problem with this claim is that, though there may be likenesses between Jenner's vaccination and what Pasteur saw happen to the chickens, there are also a number of differences. (This is an observation that the weak view of the mistake in likeness arguments makes in the case of mental illness.) Chicken cholera inoculation involves vaccination with a disease against *itself*, whereas what Jenner had observed among milk maids was protection against one disease by contracting *another*. And there are more obvious differences; in Pasteur's case we are dealing with chickens, not people, with chicken cholera and not cowpox and smallpox. Moreover, we see that these differences appear within the features that the general kind identifies. The general concept or kind is: inoculation with disease against disease; but the two specific examples are of inoculation with one disease against another and inoculation with a mild dose of a disease against itself. The general concept has to ignore these differences, or produce a description in which they disappear.

However, now we find that the likenesses that we were to suppose Pasteur observed and from which he is supposed to have reached his conclusion are being produced by the general concept, rather than the general concept being inferred from the likenesses. Inoculation against disease by disease is created by Pasteur. Things have ended up quite the other way around from what we might have expected if we thought that observation must explain what happened. In fact, Pasteur far from seeing likenesses between Jenner's vaccination and what happened to his chickens, is creating a concept in which likenesses between the two can appear (see also Soskice, 1989, p. 62).

In short this is an example of the human imagination at work through the use of metaphor. Something is being created, something that was not there previously. Moreover, this is exactly what we would expect if the strong view of the mistake in likeness arguments applied here. The likenesses appear in the light of the assignment of kind, not the other way around. We go beyond the weak view of the mistake in likeness arguments, which states that we have to do more than notice likenesses and differences, but must decide to interpret the likenesses in a particular way. Pasteur says what happened to Jenner's milk maids and his chickens can be seen in terms of vaccination; and it is in virtue of their being of the same kind that the likenesses appear between the two.

Metaphor, the strong view, and internal relations

In this subsection and the one following, I shall attempt to show that what I have said about Pasteur's chickens and the notion of vaccination is equivalent to what I earlier said about the strong view of the mistake in likeness arguments. As I have already stated, I see the strong view of the mistake in likeness arguments as the correct one in the case of mental illness. The strong view of this mistake leaves us with the question what recategorizing schizophrenia or other so-called mental illnesses comes to, and how doing so produces in these conditions the features it does. My answer will be that it comes to the use of

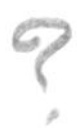

the human imagination expressed in metaphor. The features appear as a result of the internal relations between the category into which the condition is placed and the models of things which that categorization makes possible or legitimates. We shall revisit some of the earlier arguments as a result. In particular, in the next subsection, we shall revisit the argument that the illness-like features of alcoholism, ADHD, and schizophrenia are created in those conditions to the extent they are thought to be illnesses.

The analysis offered so far of Pasteur and his chickens is neat. Inevitably, potentially complicating factors do exist. Indeed, an objection clearly exists to it. I have argued that the general concept vaccination is instantiated in the particular cases if we overlook the fact that Jenner's vaccination involves different diseases and Pasteur's chickens involves the same disease. It has to pay attention instead to the idea that diseases are involved in both cases. But this was, of course, a commonplace of Pasteur's time as of ours. Why, then, should I argue that Pasteur could have noticed the differences among cowpox, smallpox, and chicken cholera, and had deliberately to ignore these to create vaccination? Surely Pasteur would simply have worked with the existing categorization here.

This objection points out that some of the various likenesses and differences between Jenner's vaccination and Pasteur's chickens pre-exist Pasteur's exclamation. So, all that seems to be missing in moving from likenesses to an attribution of kind is the decision to emphasize certain likenesses and ignore certain differences and allot to the similarities the role of making things of the same kind. This is the *weak* version of the objection to likeness arguments. A pre-existing likeness is emphasized: that smallpox, cowpox, and chicken cholera are diseases. A pre-existing difference is overlooked: that these are diseases of different kinds of creature (chickens and people) and that vaccination originally involved protection against one disease by inoculation with another. The emphasized likeness is then deemed to be a likeness that determines that what happened to the chickens shall be a kind of vaccination.

The objection is that when we attempt to criticize the use of the likeness argument in the case of vaccination and Pasteur's chickens, the argument proves incomplete, but not circular. We have to add something to complete the move from the likenesses to the conclusion. However, we do not find the conclusion contained in the very existence of the likenesses itself. It is the weak and not the strong view of the mistake in likeness arguments that Pasteur's chickens appear to lend weight to. If Pasteur is using a metaphor, then metaphor may as well be found in the weak view as in the strong. Yet I have being trying to show how it is equivalent to the strong view. The objection is that I have failed.

However, part of my problem here arises from concentrating on one element of the notion of vaccination as Pasteur created it. If we take the whole description (the protection against disease by the inoculation of disease) we do not find that this matches a pre-existing description. Likewise, the notions mental and illness pre-exist the notion of mental illness, but the combination into a new whole is what matters. Though the elements of vaccination exist separately already, the concept as a whole does not. And it is the concept as a whole that is internally related to the description of specific instances of vaccination.

The important notion here is that of *internal relation* (see Foot, 1978, particularly pp. 113ff). My claim is that the choice of description that Pasteur applies is internally related to the kind under which the events seen by him and those first witnessed by Jenner fall. The choice of a description that emphasizes that all are diseases is internally related to the description of vaccination. This ensures the circularity of the argument, which is a mark of the strong view's objection to likeness arguments. Some parts of the description of the events that vaccination, as created by Pasteur, requires were probably available already. However, their use in this case comes with Pasteur's categorization of the two events. It is when Pasteur categorizes the events in the way he does that the description comes to apply to them.

Pasteur makes what happens to the chickens vaccination. It is not something he has noticed or is reporting on. What can be said of what happened to the chickens is decided by what sort of thing is thought to have happened to them. The description in this case appears in virtue of the internal relation between it and the category of vaccination. And the category of vaccination itself involves a novel description.

Attention deficit hyperactivity disorder, alcoholism, schizophrenia, and the strong view revisited

The introduction of the notion of internal relation at this juncture needs to be applied retrospectively to the earlier arguments about the existence of genetic causation in the case of ADHD (and in the case of alcoholism as is sometimes proposed), and of dysfunction in the case of schizophrenia. In the case of the chickens we can allow that some features of likeness between chicken cholera and Jenner's vaccination existed in virtue of internal relations other than that of Pasteur's vaccination. Smallpox, cowpox, and chicken cholera are all diseases, but not because they are gathered under the heading of vaccination. The same could be true with the features of ADHD (and of alcoholism). It is possible that ADHD and alcoholism could be described as genetically predisposed without being described as illnesses.

This would be the case if, for instance, someone were to take the line that there is an element of genetic predisposition in all or much of our behaviour—and not only in behaviour such as ADHD or alcoholism but also in behaviour such as going to football matches. True, there is a connection between describing ADHD or alcoholism as illnesses and what we think the features of ADHD and alcoholism are or will be found to be. If we describe them as illnesses then we will no doubt start to think in terms of genetic predisposition, and set up research programmes to identify the genes that are responsible for this (as in the case of Smith–Magenis syndrome). However, this may be true of any categorization of the human condition we call ADHD or alcoholism provided only the categorization in question may imply that sort of feature. If we hold that we are genetically predisposed to all or at least many of our human behaviours, going to football matches will be described in these terms, and ADHD and alcoholism will be too. However, we will not be seen as genetically predisposed to ADHD or alcoholism in virtue of their being illnesses, but in virtue only of their being behaviours. ADHD and alcoholism will take this description in virtue of their internal relation to the category behaviours rather than because of their internal relation to the category illness.

This does not, however, destroy the position the strong view takes up with regard to ADHD or alcoholism. Plainly we do not have to describe ADHD or alcoholism as behaviours with a genetic predisposition, as that description is patently controversial. (Or, to put the point another way, what we mean by genetic predisposition may be nothing to do with cause; this was a point we considered in Chapter 2.) However, our choice of description of the features of ADHD or alcoholism is determined by, or internally related to, what kind of thing we think they are none the less. What we cannot necessarily conclude from the mere existence of the claim that people are genetically predisposed to ADHD or alcoholism, is that illness is the more general kind under which they are being included. We do not need to suggest that the existence of this internal connection excludes all other internal connections between ADHD and alcoholism and other categories by which we explain and understand the world around us. It may be claimed that internal relations to one category do exclude internal relations to another. It might be argued, as we shall see, that you cannot hold that ADHD and/or alcoholism are behaviours and that they are illnesses (this is the burden of the sort of scepticism we have been considering over the past chapters). However, the strong argument need only demonstrate that the choice of descriptions is internally related to some assignment of kind; and that the assignment of kind implies certain descriptions. Individual things may be internally related to a number of kinds.

Behaviour, illness, and internal relations

I have just now mentioned that describing ADHD or alcoholism as a behaviour to which we may be predisposed by our genes does not necessarily lead to the conclusion that either condition is being described as an illness. It may be that they are being described as behaviours, along with going to football matches and all sorts of other activities, by someone who holds that all behaviour exhibits an element of genetic predisposition. However, I have also canvassed the possibility that describing something in terms internally related to one kind or category may rule out describing it in terms internally related to another category. For example I argued that someone objecting to the existence of the category mental illness might argue that illnesses should be described in natural terms (in terms for example of dysfunctions and causes) while behaviour should be described in moral, social, and political terms. These are the two sets of descriptive resources that Latour (1993) observed in the discourse of Boyle and Hobbes over the question of the existence in nature of a vacuum, and which he thinks represent the enlightenment dualism of the natural and the social. The possibility that things can be described in one set or terms or in the other, but not both, is worth further consideration.

We earlier asked how we are to explain the occurrences that we call by the name schizophrenia, and consist of complex bizarre beliefs. (Frith (1992) mentions believing that one's thoughts are being broadcast or someone else's thoughts are being inserted into one's brain. Szasz (1982) mentions the belief that one is being pursued by communists or that one is Napoleon.) One possible explanation is subtle brain disease. My claim, consistent with the strong view, is that there is an internal relation between the belief that schizophrenia is a subtle brain disease and the features that we take schizophrenia to show. We can use our imagination to see such complex bizarre beliefs in these terms; and in doing so we create the features of schizophrenia that go with that way of seeing it.

Indeed, Szasz presents the sort of case which might be made to support just such a version of what does happen in the case of mental illness. Speaking of the communications given by schizophrenics about themselves (such as 'I am being pursued by communists' or 'I am Napoleon') and explanations in terms of brain disease, Szasz says: 'Explanations of this sort of occurrence—assuming that one is interested in the belief itself and does not regard it simply as a "symptom" or expression of something else that is *more interesting*—must be sought along different lines.' (1982, p. 20, Szasz's italics).

If we omit the passage between the dashes, we get Szasz's argument that there can be no such thing as mental illness: 'Explanations of this sort of occurrence . . . *must* be sought along different lines' (my italics), i.e. on lines other than that of subtle brain disease. But if we include the passage between the dashes the word must becomes conditional upon the kind of interest we take in a schizophrenic's communications. The suggestion here seems to be that we can take a variety of interests in the apparent phenomena of schizophrenia. We can take the sort of interest that we take in beliefs in general. Or we can look behind or beyond the beliefs to something else of which they are merely an expression or symptom (see also Smith, 1978, pp. 37–8).

Szasz, in this passage, does not say that we *cannot* be interested in a human phenomenon as a symptom of something else, something else we find more interesting. (This is what he should say if he wanted to hold that mental illness must be conceptually confused.) What Szasz does say is that to be interested *in the belief itself* is to be interested in the occurrence in a particular way. Being interested in the occurrence in that way excludes the idea that the belief is not actually a belief at all, but a symptom (of a subtle brain disease for example). Szasz is saying, in effect, that there is a *conceptual* disjunction between seeing something as a belief and seeing it as a symptom. You can see in a schizophrenic's report about herself either a complex bizarre belief or a symptom. Szasz holds that these are conceptually exclusive options. You cannot have it both ways; schizophrenia cannot without contradiction be described in terms internally related to both. However, he does not say (here) that you can take only one kind of interest. He merely points out that the kind of interest you take and the kind of thing you take what you see to be are interconnected. And this is precisely what the strong view contends. And this is precisely what metaphors represent happening: taking something to be one kind of thing rather than another.

Szasz's notion that taking the kind of interest we take in behaviour excludes taking the kind of interest we take in symptoms and disease can be countered. An alcoholic's drinking may be regarded as motivated, perhaps by the need to forget or escape or for hedonistic reasons. In this sense, the alcoholic's actions may be regarded as behaviour, in being undertaken for a reason. This would distinguish them from actions seen as symptoms that would perhaps appear in contrast as puppet like. At the same time, the motivations themselves may be regarded as ill. These, medicine may appropriately take an interest in.

Szasz would no doubt reply that to see motivations as ill is to redescribe them in such a way that they are no longer motivations as we usually think of them: for example, they become symptomatic themselves. However, my position does not require me to resolve this issue in either direction. In fact, the claims I have been making are confirmed by the existence of such disputes. We can deny that physical features of the brain or brain chemistry must force us into calling any human condition associated with them an illness, disease, or disorder. This is because the actual relation between the physical features of the brain and the behaviours, motivations, attitudes, beliefs, and other mental states and events within a person, can always be described in ways that do not imply illness. In Szasz's terms we can take more than one kind of interest in the phenomena. The same terms apply equally well to alcoholism, ADHD, and schizophrenia. In the case of alcoholism, the correlation of alpha waves may interest as causing disease insofar as causal connections of this kind are medical notions; the person's failure to resist the lure of the pleasures of alcohol may interest us as a case of moral weakness in the face of temptation. In the case of ADHD, a genetic correlation may interest us as evidence of disease or illness insofar as a genetic predisposition is a medical notion; the person's failure to concentrate on tough but important school or other work may interest us as a case of weakness of purpose in the face of distraction. In the case of schizophrenia, having highly abnormal beliefs may interest us as a pointer to some dysfunction of the mind or brain; it may interest us as other ordinary beliefs do, for its content and consistency or for the care someone has taken to check its validity. The question of whether a feature of the brain related to a human condition turns that condition into an illness of any sort is in part a matter of the kind of interest we take in it.

We can associate these different forms of interest with the two halves of the dualism Latour imputes to the moderns. To take an interest in a person's behaviours is to take an interest in them as products of society. That is to say, it is to take an interest in them in terms of the social meanings that behaviours may have. This is where notions of intention, attitude, and value come in. Behaviours exist in the light of such ideas—such ideas are internally related to what we think of as behaviour. On the other hand, to take an interest in underlying causes of actions is to take an interest in them as the products of nature. That is to say, it is to take an interest in them in terms of the relations between the structures, functions, and forces in terms of which we understand human biology. These ideas are internally related to what we think of as illness. As Latour (1993) noted, the moderns tend to think of these two sets of descriptive resources as mutually exclusive. They believed in them as pure: things fit into either one kind of description or the other.

Latour, as I have earlier indicated, is not satisfied with this. He says the purification never really happens. The modernist purification is an artificiality. He introduces, instead, the idea of hybrid objects. These are objects that we can describe as existing where many different forms of interest intersect. We earlier considered Latour's account of the hybrid object the ozone hole. And we developed an example in which schizophrenia might be the hybrid object. In any of the examples of mental illnesses we have considered—ADHD and alcoholism, for example—a similar story involving multiple forms of interest (in things as natural and as social at once) can be told. That is to say, the idea that things are either one or the other is, to Latour, mistaken. Hence, Latour implicitly rejects the idea that the two forms of description are exclusive, at least in the sense that objects can fall under only one or the other, and not both.

Broadly speaking, I think Latour is right. For example, it may well be that, at one and the same time, alcoholism is held to be a behaviour and an illness. This would be in true in the sense that in any case involving alcoholism, there may be numerous different issues, social and medical, mixed up. For example, it may be held that the availability and popularity of drink is part of the problem. The person who becomes an alcoholic lives in a world in which alcohol may be well accepted, and drinking to excess may be seen as the cool thing to do. Evidence of both of these is to be had in the bars around the university campus I teach on Friday and Saturday nights. So part of what we understand by alcoholism may be related to the high value placed upon alcohol. But at the same time, a genetic causal account can be entertained. Different branches of our health services may proceed at the same time on these two aspects of the understanding of alcoholism. Preventive measures may be directed at social attitudes to drink and drunkenness: therapeutic measures may be directed at individuals.

However, though Latour may be right, what still remains true is that none of these descriptive possibilities force themselves upon us. A sceptic about alcoholism does not have to accept a story in terms of the causal role of genes; a non-sceptic does not have to accept a story in terms of moral failures, of either the individual or society. This is parallel to the case with Pasteur and vaccination.

Nothing he saw forced upon him the idea that what happened to the chickens was vaccination. Any description given of these events that draws attention to the likenesses that the notion of vaccination makes possible, is an attempt to say how what Pasteur saw and what Jenner saw are alike given they are of the same kind. The metaphor baldly states that they are of the same kind, and does no more. The description works within the possibilities that metaphor creates. Of course, this is not to say that similarities are the only possibility metaphor creates. We might equally talk about the differences between things of the same kind, or of differences within certain shared features of things, such as differences of colour, size, or significance. Metaphors, as Davidson (1984) rightly suggests, do not constrain or dictate our descriptions or thoughts.

5.3 The body is a machine

The example of Pasteur's chickens is localized. As an instance of the use of the creative imagination it is significant, but the creativity in this case is restricted in application. I want now to look at the idea that the body is a machine, an example where the application is itself extremely wide; as wide as the whole spectrum of disease and illness on some accounts, and perhaps as wide as modern medicine itself. In the idea that the body is a machine we have an internal relation between the features of a thing—the body—and the kind of thing we think the body is on a grand scale.

Boorse (e.g. 1977) and Wakefield (1992a, b) seem to grant the metaphor this conceptual breadth through their attitude to the notion of dysfunction. Boorse holds that disease is dysfunction; Wakefield holds that disorder is necessarily a dysfunction. They use these ideas as a basis for arguing that mental disease (disorder) exists. Their arguments are that we can see that conditions such as schizophrenia reveal dysfunctions, that dysfunction and disease (disorder) are closely related concepts, and that to that extent schizophrenia is a disease (or can be a disorder).

The idea that medical terms such as disease and disorder involve dysfunction is consistent with the outlook of some modern anatomy textbooks. Here we find the idea that the human body is a functioning structure—a machine. This idea is also quite familiar to the lay person. The heart is often spoken of as pumping the blood around the body, the brain is sometimes said to be a computer, and the lungs a kind of bellows. It comes naturally, perhaps, to us in the later part of the twentieth century to think of the parts and systems of the body in these terms. *Gray's Anatomy* (Williams *et al.*, 1989) bases its account of the human anatomy on the proposition that the body is a functioning structure. I quote from the introduction:

> ... all functions occur in structures and the basic medical discipline, anatomy, necessarily provides a basis for all functional studies. But the anatomist may, and often does, stop the machine, describing it, even ad nauseam, without

> appeal to its function. This policy, though fortunately not often nowadays pursued to the ultimate, deprives the subject of its content of rationality. It is difficult to imagine investigation of a structure without a concomitant desire to elucidate function, development or any other aspects of structure. Long ago Descartes described man as a complex of machinery—bio-chemical, micro- and macro-anatomical—and machines work; all *living* structures are constantly changing at one level or another. Williams *et al.* (1989, p. 3)

This way of speaking and thinking is not abnormal or unnatural for us. Nevertheless, I shall suggest that there is a metaphor here. That metaphor is contained in the idea that humans are a 'complex of machinery' or, more simply, the body is a machine. *Gray's* identifies an historical point at which this idea became current, that is in the early seventeenth century in the work of René Descartes. Though Descartes is said to have described humans 'as a complex of machinery', and the word as is associated with simile, the implication of the passage is stronger than the idea that the body is like a machine. It is closer to saying people's bodies are machines than to saying it is *as if* they are machines.

It is in its more detailed anatomical description that *Gray's* use of the idea that the body is a machine goes further than saying 'the body is like a machine'.

> As in most musical instruments, the mechanism of speech consists of three essentials: a source of energy, structures capable of periodic and aperiodic oscillations and a resonator. Energy is derived from the velocity of the expired air, oscillation primarily from the vocal folds and resonance from the multiform 'column' of air extending from the folds to the lips and nostrils. Williams *et al.* (1989, p. 1257)

And so on. Together with the accompanying diagrams, the text seeks to describe the human vocal organs entirely in terms of their structural anatomy and functions.

We shall return to this passage from *Gray's* in Chapter 8. There we shall discuss the difference between the metaphor 'the body is a machine' and the specific models it makes possible (the human vocal organs are like a musical instrument). We will find that the description given here of the vocal organs as a musical instrument could in theory be countered, by a more effective machine analogy or model. The actual descriptions that become possible of the body—the actual models that may be used—once it is said to be a machine will depend very much on what machines exist, and how their workings are described. These possibilities are contingent upon history, developments in science and technology outside medicine, and so on.

This is not to say that metaphor is not an historical event: I have already argued that it is. Rather it is to point out that the metaphor 'the body is a machine' does not determine what descriptions will be given of the parts of the body. All that is determined by the metaphor is that a certain kind of description of the body shall be possible. And this kind of description takes over the whole body. As *Gray's* description suggests, the mechanical facts we appeal to about the body, as it were occupy the whole body. The body has become categorized with other machines. In the history of medicine, there came a time when these facts invaded the body, while the previous set of facts about the body were evicted, lock, stock, and barrel. The kind of facts that occupy the space of the body come with the general way of looking at the body. The general way of looking at the body is a question of how the body is classified or categorized. What we see in the body, what features we take it to have, what analogies we are prepared to countenance or work out, come with, and are dependent upon this classification or categorization.

It follows that we cannot find facts about the body that will enable us to dispute whether or not it is a machine. Given that the facts that occupy the space of the body come and go all together, they cannot help mediate between different ways of looking at the body. Nor could such facts test different ways of looking at the body. The very facts we may appeal to appear as facts about the body only in the light of the way we look at the body; the way we look at the body does not appear in the light of the facts about it. The category into which the body is fitted is not determined by the body's features: the body's features are determined by the category into which it is fitted. And this is parallel to what the strong view claims in the case of mental illness: the likenesses between two human conditions or between a part of the body and some machine appear in virtue of descriptions of those things, and these descriptions depend upon what kind of thing they are thought to be. Metaphor simply refers to the imaginative moving of something into a category (schizophrenia into the category of illness, the body into the category of machine).

It is clear that we do not have to think of the whole body in mechanical terms. That is to say the body does not have to be fitted into the category of machines. History teaches us that this view arrived with the scientific revolution of the seventeenth century. Some suggest that the metaphor 'the body is a machine', at least as machines were conceived by Descartes, has been under critical scrutiny from within Western science since the late nineteenth century (Verwy, 1990, p. 140). Cultural studies tell us that even today systems of medicine flourish, which take a quite different view of the organs of the human body.

More generally, some may say that to think of the body as a machine entails forgetting that each human body is not merely a body but also a person (Cassell, 1991, especially p. 49; Wulff, 1994). There is scope for disagreement, then. In seeing human bodies, which are only a part of the whole person, as machines, we may bring together ideas that, to some at any rate, seem to come from different worlds. To these people the idea that the body is a machine is an incoherent combination of ideas, or perhaps represents quite the wrong sort of interest to take in it.

Because the idea that the body is a machine is so entrenched in the basic medical sciences such as anatomy, the thought that it may be challenged is potentially a radical one. Perhaps it is even more radical than Szasz's challenge to psychiatry. However, the two challenges rest on the same sort of footing. They both entail the claim that the categorization involved is wrong. That is to say, they both involve the rejection of a metaphor.

Conclusions

The notion of metaphor developed in the previous chapter, has been taken up in this. In two examples I have tried to show how an act of the imagination may create the objects of science. The two cases stand at opposite ends of a range. Pasteur's claims about vaccination are significant, but they are localized. They do not represent a wholesale change in ways of looking at things. They represent a development in or creation of a category. This development appears relatively uncontroversial. The claim that the body is a machine, whether made by Descartes in the early seventeenth century, or the editors of *Gray's Anatomy* in the late twentieth century, is a claim of a different order of magnitude. It underlies a shift in vision profound and embracing enough almost to be classified as a world view (to take up Stephen Pepper's (1961) terminology). It has spawned an almost numberless clutch of succeeding analogies and explanations.

The next part of the book explores the idea that mental illness is no more and no less a metaphor than is the idea that the body is a machine. It looks into the history of the emergence of mental illness and of ADHD in order to see the metaphor at work, much as, in the chapter, we have looked into history to see other metaphors at work.

Sceptics such as Szasz will have none of this. To him metaphor is a loose cannon. It appears to build bridges between things, or team things up, in ways in which they really cannot be teamed up. What remarkable things we can do with language, in poetry for example, is free of danger, because free of sequelae. If thoughts may be green, plans cast-iron, memories distant, and so forth, in verse or in our day-to-day talk, that is fine. But poets, contrary to what Shelley (1947, p. 59) said, should not legislate what the world is like; language should not have a hand in making the world. Problems arise when the kind of imagination we find so enthralling and inspiring in poetry is let loose in science. No good, Szasz believes, can come of that.

But Szasz is wrong. Metaphor is linked to the capacity of the human imagination to create new categories, or to recategorize things. In these imaginative leaps, the features of the world do not remain unchanged, but are altered. There is a very real sense in which we make the body a machine; in which Pasteur made what happened to his chickens into vaccination. These notions are to be found in the heartland of physical medical science. Yet Szasz seeks to contrast psychiatry with physical medicine. I shall argue we make schizophrenia or alcoholism or ADHD into illnesses and hence make mental illness in much the same way we make the body into a machine. The chapters of the next part of the book seek to set out this argument, explore it in a number of different contexts, and to justify it against a number of objections.

Endnotes

1 From Latin *vaccinus* (= vaccine) meaning 'cow pox virus' from Latin *vacca* meaning 'cow' (Allen, 1990).

2 Lawrie Reznek would I think take issue with Szasz on this point. He holds (1991, pp. 74ff) that this is evidence of Szasz's dualism, and Reznek thinks that dualism is a mistaken account of the relation of mind and body. Reznek believes that we can correctly talk about our reasonable beliefs being caused, by the evidence for them, for example. So he rejects the idea that causes and reasons exclude one another. This is not the place to go into the question of whether Reznek is right, even supposing I had the philosophical knowledge to do so. I can only flag up two problems I have with his account. First, it seems to me that Szasz can accept talk of causes for beliefs provided that directs us towards things like evidence and so forth. What I would want to resist, on Szasz's behalf, is any move to say beliefs apparently inadequately supported by evidence have to be looked at in a different way (as something to do with illness and all that entails). Second, Reznek thinks that he can give an account of the relation between the mind and the body, and supposes that Szasz must be doing so too. Reznek's account is monist (he holds that mind and body are identical); while Szasz's, he thinks, must be dualist. Reznek assumes that 'the mind' is a single thing standing in a single relationship to the body. When Szasz says that 'the mind' is an abstract noun that refers to a whole collection of things he does not seem to me committed to this assumption. In that sense, I do not think Szasz is necessarily a dualist: he may regard the whole question of *the* relation of mind to body as improperly formulated. Dualism, and monism, as supposed responses to this improper question would likewise be improper.

Part 3

The metaphor of mental illness

6 The metaphor of mental illness

6.1 Introduction

The three chapters in this third section of the book take up the notion of metaphor discussed and illustrated in Section 2, and apply it in the case of mental illness. Emerging in the first two of the three chapters is a difficulty in the position I am advancing. This difficulty is that it is very close to positions that are sceptical about the existence of mental illness (or about the illness status of particular patterns or claimed patterns of behaviour such as those designated by ADHD). The difficulty arises because the role I assign to metaphor is so very fundamental. I assert that the categorization as mental illness of claimed patterns of behaviour such as those referred to by diagnoses of schizophrenia, alcoholism, and ADHD happens by metaphor. They are shifted from one sphere of explanation and understanding—that offered in social, political, moral terms—and into another sphere of explanation and understanding—that offered in medical terms—by an imaginative categorization.

The implication of this is that psychiatry creates the objects of its investigations, its diagnosis and treatment, in the light of its own approach. But this seems to be the basis of damaging criticism of psychiatry: creating the objects of investigation is one mark of what is sometimes called pseudo-science. One expects genuine sciences, on the other hand, to be investigations into objects that exist in nature—which do not have to be created by the scientists or by the wider society. We can express the distinction in the language that we used earlier to distinguish the descriptive resources that seem to be available in the case of illness from those that refer to the mental. One would expect a genuine object of medical science to be a natural object: something that is not made by humans.

In the case of illness this point needs to be clarified slightly. Many illnesses are the result of human activity: for example, they may be said to result from human lifestyle, diet, or work conditions. Lack of exercise, fast food, and pollution may all be blamed for causing diseases. Diseases that result from these are indeed the creation of people. However, such diseases, though created by humans in this sense, are not the creations of human in the sense in which I claim that mental illness is the creation of humans. Diseases that result from the activities of humans can still be instantiated in the natural (biological or psychological) fabric of the individual. As such, they are identifiable in terms such as dysfunction or lesion, which refer to this biological/psychological fabric. In this sense, they are not created by people. And this is the sense I use when I say that illness seems to be a natural object.

Of course, the specific understandings and theories about such objects (e.g. mental illnesses) have to be created by people, that is to say the scientists. However, this is quite different from saying that the objects themselves are created by the scientists. To say that the objects are created in the same way as the theories about them would make those objects into the kinds of thing that we associate with society as opposed to those we associate with the natural: values, ideas, beliefs, and so on. These things are made by society or by groups within society.

The difficulty my position threatens to get into is that it appears to show that psychiatry is a pseudo-science—which is just what the sceptical approach claimed it was. The difficulty may be expressed in rather different ways. In this chapter, where I consider the development of the notion of mental illness in the nineteenth century, the difficulty appears in a parallel between my analysis and the analysis offered by the strong programme in the sociology of knowledge. This programme holds that the objects of scientific knowledge are reproductions of social objects—specifically the categories into which people are organized. This suggests that the supposed natural objects of scientific investigation are actually nothing of the sort. In the next chapter, where I turn to a twentieth/twenty-first century example, namely ADHD, the difficulty appears in the parallel between my account and that of the social constructionist. The social constructionist, at least as I interpret his/her position, holds that ADHD exists only in certain cultural or social frames of reference. The social constructionist also claims that what appears to be a natural object—what is presented as made by the hand of nature rather than by humans—will prove to be a social object (an idea) created in virtue of social beliefs.

My position seems to be threatened with the difficulty of distinguishing itself from scepticism because in both these cases what a sceptic about mental illness might say is that the imaginative recategorization represents the point at which what are in fact social and political ideas become transmuted into what they are not—medical ideas. Moreover, there seems, particularly in the case of the social constructionist's analysis of such things as ADHD, to be an implication of deceit—just what sceptic Thomas Szasz says is part of metaphor. However, in both cases I'd want to say we neither have such a transmutation, nor necessarily any deception.

6.2 Madness and mental illness in nineteenth century Britain

Marking the end of a period of historical revolution for the notion of madness or insanity, David Pilgrim (1992, p. 211) points out an 1858 editorial in the *Journal of Mental Science* (forerunner of the *British Journal of Psychiatry*) that declares: 'Insanity is purely a disease of the brain. The physician is now the responsible guardian of the lunatic and must ever remain so'. What this revolution in the status of the concept meant socially and politically is summed up by Scull in these terms:

> Insanity had been transformed from a vague, culturally defined phenomenon affecting an unknown, but probably small, proportion of the population into a condition that could be authoritatively diagnosed, certified, and dealt with only by a group of legally recognized experts and that was now seen as one of the major forms of deviance in English society. . . . with the achievement of what is conventionally called 'lunacy reform,' the asylum was endorsed as the sole officially approved response to the problems posed by mental illness. Throughout the length and breadth of the country, huge specialized buildings had been built or were in the process of being built to accommodate the legions of the mad. Scull (1989, p. 216)

Scull does not employ the notion of metaphor to describe how this recategorization and expansion of insanity was achieved. And of course statements such as 'Insanity is purely a disease of the brain' can be interpreted in more than one way. A non-metaphorical construal would be that these words describe a discovery about insanity, perhaps supporting the sort of hypothesis William Cullen advanced as early as 1785. He postulated that certain mental disorders were the result of some unknown physical change in the nerves, for which he coined the term neurosis. This term has since quite altered its meaning, as it now refers not to a state of the nerves but to a nervous state. If the editor of the *Journal of Mental Science* is not referring to a discovery, he may still be referring to a hypothesis, though one which can be asserted with considerable certainty. In both cases, it appears possible to take the statement as being a factual statement about what is taken to be a factual matter.

However, the statement that madness is 'purely a disease of the brain' need be factual only in the sense that 'the body is a machine' is factual. That is to say, it need not represent a statement about how the world organizes itself. It may rather represent a metaphor: the wrong categorization of insanity by means of wrong naming.

What would a sceptic about mental illness (such as Szasz) say had happened in the nineteenth century in the UK to lead to the revolution of which Scull and Pilgrim speak? Szasz implies that psychiatry takes up the terminology of a genuine science (medicine) and imposes it in a place where it becomes a pseudo-science (psychiatry). These are not his words, but I think his arguments tend towards this conclusion. Mental illness is a metaphor; the science of psychiatry is based upon it; so, if psychiatry is a science in any sense, it is in a metaphorical (or a pseudo) sense.

We can state the view of the scientific status of psychiatry implicit in a sceptical approach such as that of Szasz in the following terms: Psychiatry cannot be a science since it has no scientific object. Sciences are interested in the objective features of objective things; but so-called mental illnesses are not fundamentally different in their objective state from sanity. By the phrase objective state in the medical sciences the sceptical approach understands such things as physical anatomical or physical or mental functional correlates to illness experiences. In physical disease, our subjective experience of the difficulty of breathing may correlate with the inflammation of the lining of our lungs. This inflammation is itself an abnormal state of the lungs in anatomical terms. It can be identified quite apart from the undesired and unpleasant experience of wheezing and coughing. However, the sceptical approach believes we will be unable to tell the physical and functional correlates of those said to be mentally ill from those said to be mentally healthy if we look at those correlates alone.

That is not to say that we cannot distinguish a group of behaviours that we may call schizophrenic, depressive, ADHD, or alcoholic, from other groups of behaviours (though Boyle (1990) argues that we have not in the case of schizophrenia). We distinguish between types of behaviour all the time. We do so on broadly social and ethical grounds; behaviours can be impolite, impolitic, impious, and impossible. However, it could be said, these are not the sort of grounds upon which a genuine medical scientific distinction could be made. This is because impolite behaviour—rudeness, to pick an example at random—is not an objective fact or feature of a behaviour. Instead it is a social judgement about behaviour; or we can say it is the socially created meaning of the behaviour. The point is that there can be no scientific, that is to say, no objective basis in the anatomical distinctions of diseased and healthy, or in distinctions between what is dysfunctional and what functional, for a distinction of a social and ethical sort such as rudeness. A rude person may be in rude health. And by the same token, any genuine scientific distinction among human behaviours will inevitably be blind to the ethical status our beliefs place upon those behaviours.

However, the sceptic argues, psychiatry cannot help but call upon our social and ethical attitudes, because it inevitably starts from the identification of certain patterns of behaviour (something that appears rather obvious when one looks at taxonomies of mental illness such as the American Psychiatric Association's *Diagnostic and Statistical Manual of Mental Disorders*). To the behaviours identified in these non-scientific terms it appears to apply a series of objective medical notions. But this is, the sceptic argues, merely an appearance. The application is metaphorical through and through. The behaviours, the sceptical approach says, do not have objective physical (or psychological) features to which the medical terms could refer. In particular, behaviours cannot be distinguished by means of the medical terms diseased or ill.

With physical illness the case, for the sceptical approach, is quite different. This, it says, is objectively differentiable from healthy conditions. Physical illness involves changes in the structures of the body, or the functioning of organs of the body, describable in terms of the sciences of anatomy and physiology. That someone is ill is not, for the sceptic, a social or a moral judgement, and does not rely upon one. Rather, it is an anatomical or physiological judgement, arising from the descriptive resources of the medical science of anatomy.

The sceptic is implying a more general contrast—one I shall be particularly concerned with in the remainder of this chapter, and one that closely reflects a distinction we discussed in earlier chapters—the distinction between things that are the product of nature and things that are the product of society or some group or section of society. On the one side there are sciences such as anatomy and medicine, but presumably also physics, chemistry, and biology; and on the other pseudo-sciences such as psychiatry, but presumably also alchemy, phrenology and other discredited endeavours. The mark of the pseudo-science is that it is responsible for the creation of the object it claims to have identified and to be exploring or explaining. Szasz, for example (1979, p. 9, cited in Reznek, 1991, pp. 76–7) says that Kraepelin and Bleuler 'did not discover [dementia praecox and schizophrenia] . . . they invented them'. Boyle says that 'psychiatrists behave *as if* they were studying bodily functioning and *as if* they had described patterns there, when in fact they are studying behaviour' (Boyle, 1990, p. 179). Breggin, who is a sceptic about ADHD and whose views will be looked at in the next chapter, says that psychiatrists always see things in psychiatric terms, even when (as he contends is the case in ADHD) they have no scientific basis for doing so (Breggin, 1998, p. 173). The sceptic's claim is that psychiatry creates the things it studies (for example schizophrenia) by evaluating things according to ethical or other social norms (i.e. as behaviour). The mark of a science seems, by contrast, to be the fact that its object has an existence independent of human evaluation and norms. At any rate, it has an existence independent of social, moral, or religious values (cf. Boyle, 1990, p. 92). Physical disease and physical medicine exist in virtue of the norms of anatomy and/or physiology. However, according to the sceptical position, the same claims cannot be made on behalf of mental illness or psychiatry.

So, to determine whether something is a pseudo or merely metaphorical science, in sceptical terms, we have to find out whether the scientists and/or elements in wider society are creating the objects in question themselves. We have to find whether the things in question—in our case the mental illnesses—exist independently of the interests and values of the psychiatrists and the society in which they flourish. In short, to show to a sceptic's satisfaction that psychiatry is a genuine science we would have to show that mental illness exists in virtue of the application of medical terms. And the sceptic says that when we do apply these terms as they should be applied, we do not end up with mental illnesses at all. We can get to so-called mental illness only by applying another set of terms—those that originate with our values. The so-called mental illnesses are collections of behaviours that people disvalue in one way and another. People find schizophrenics bizarre, their claims wild, their behaviour unmanageable and frightening. That is how schizophrenia is identified. However, this does not separate the identification from the values of the identifiers. To do that some medical correlate would need to be found. For the sceptic the behaviour of schizophrenics is not medically anatomically (or functionally) distinct from the behaviour of members of small religious cults; and nor is it anatomically (functionally) distinct from his or her own behaviour. That is to say, from within the resources of anatomy or psychology no correlating distinction of healthy and unhealthy will be possible.

Someone may ask how a sceptic, such as Szasz, can be so clear about these claims. They look as if they may be empirical claims; that is, claims made upon the basis of experimental research into the relation of neurology and behaviour, perhaps. However, the sceptic can be clear and certain because these claims are not empirical. When Szasz says 'schizophrenic symptoms are not caused by an underlying lesion' (cited Reznek, 1991, p. 77; cf. also p. 92) I would claim he is making a conceptual statement. When we speak of behaviour, Szasz says, we mean to refer to something that is distinguishable in terms of moral and social judgements and beliefs. Behaviour is internally related to these. When we speak of health and illness we mean to refer to something that is distinguishable in terms of anatomical judgements (or perhaps functional judgements—though this is something about which Szasz himself is sceptical). We cannot, then, talk about behaviours and at the same time talk about illnesses. Szasz puts it thus: 'we will discover the chemical cause of schizophrenia when we will discover the chemical cause of Judaism, Christianity, and Communism. No sooner and no later' (Szasz, 1974b, pp. 101–2; cited by Reznek, 1991, p. 74). We cannot regard these as chemically caused, as we think of them as beliefs. Szasz's implication is that we cannot discover the chemical cause of schizophrenia.

So much for what I take the sceptic to be thinking. And I go along with much of it. What I do not share is the sceptic's intended use of these points. Briefly, I have argued that *some of what there is* is determined by *how we think*. Vaccination appears in the mind of Pasteur. The machine-like properties of the body appear in the minds of seventeenth century philosophers and scientists. And, in particular, some of what may be regarded as objective medical features of conditions such as alcoholism, or schizophrenia, appear when those conditions are thought of as illnesses. In applying ADHD to the understanding and explanation of the behaviours of certain children and adults, and referring to genetic correlations as causal or predisposing, we show that we are thinking of these behaviours in illness terms.

Where precisely is the difference between a sceptic and myself? I want to hold on to the idea that psychiatry may be a science while at the same time thinking that some of the objects of the science are created by the scientists. Psychiatrists may be interested in the causal connections between the structures of the brain and the behaviours of humans such as those said to be alcoholic or to have ADHD; or they may be interested in the functional aspects of the mind in schizophrenia. However, I find that the very existence of these connections and functions depends upon the way in which the psychiatrists look at alcoholism, ADHD, and schizophrenia. The psychiatrists do indeed create the objects of their own science. Given this, how do I hope to elude a sceptical analysis of psychiatry?

My answer is double aspected: First, the invention of possible categories is precisely what we have seen Pasteur doing with vaccination; and the recategorization of something such that our possible descriptions of it are altered is precisely what happened with the body in the seventeenth century. So, plausibly, sciences other than psychiatry rely to some degree upon what humans create, but in these other cases this is not regarded as a sufficient reason for impugning their scientific basis.

Second, I hope to show that my position does not commit me to the idea that what humans create must always be created in the image of their own values, or in the image of social and political realities. There is a middle path here. We do not have to choose between a pseudo-science, which is in reality the imposition of a set of values upon an oppressed minority (the values of the Orthodox or of the psychiatrist or, as it might be put, the dominant values of society), and a science, which has to be based entirely upon categories and concepts inferred from the observable features of nature. The truth about the objects of science is that some of them lie outside these two choices; and this is why and how we can say things about psychiatry and physical medicine as sciences, while holding on to the idea that they are also reflections of the human imagination.

6.3 Mental illness and the role of the social (1)

We have identified the way in which a sceptic such as Szasz and I differ. Metaphor, for the sceptic, is a means of imposing what we might call in a broad sense values (a combination of beliefs, ideas, judgements, and so on). It drives over a merely nominal bridge, and into an area properly occupied by human behaviours, the language that properly applies to medicine. In reality, the sceptic says, this new language does not change the area it attempts to occupy. Instead, within the area of human behaviours, the same old set of social and ethical distinctions continues to be applied. However, the new language dresses some of these up as medical distinctions. Some people society does not much care for, or does not know what to do with, such as those called schizophrenics, fall under the power of psychiatrists. This is all the work of metaphor: we call (wrongly name) a social and ethical judgement an illness judgement; a schizophrenic is called (wrongly named) ill.

For me, metaphor is a means of rethinking our categorization of the world, and of creating new categories and features of the world. When the new language arrives across the nominal bridge, it does not leave things as they were. It changes some of them. Indeed, quite likely, some of the things it may change change because they were the creation of the previous language that has now been replaced.[1] This is parallel to the idea that prior to the idea that the body was a machine some other metaphor held sway. And this is not merely the imposition of a set of values by deceptive means. Deception may not be involved at all.

Despite these encouraging possible parallels, the sceptic has a number of resources to support his or her claim that there is something particularly suspect about psychiatry and mental illness. These emerge when we look in more detail at how historians relate and interpret the events of the early nineteenth century in the UK by which madness came to be medicalized. A further example will be considered in the next chapter, which revisits many of these issues in the context of ADHD looked at from a social constructionist perspective. In both cases the sceptic can point to a picture of a social and political (as I shall later call it, simply, an historical) process, and not by any means a scientific, process. It is this that, in the case of mental illness in the nineteenth century determines the development of the idea of mental illness and of the institutions of psychiatry, such as the lunatic asylums, which purported to treat and cure it or were at least set up with that aim. Likewise, it is a process of this kind that the social constructivist sees in the development of ADHD during the twentieth century.

The development of the notion of mental illness in the UK

Historians tell us that the modern concept of mental illness begins to appear in the late eighteenth and early nineteenth centuries. Thomas Szasz says this is about the same time as the modern idea of physical illness began to develop and about the time urbanization and a sense of human rights became important features (Miller and Szasz, 1983, pp. 274–5). He sometimes locates its development with the move from structural to functional diseases at the time of Charcot and later Freud (1974a, particularly chapter 2). Scull, as we shall see in more detail shortly, locates its development with the growth of market capitalism in the earlier eighteenth century (Scull, 1989).

No doubt the emergence of mental illness occurs in historically different ways in different places. My example will be that of the UK. As we saw earlier, by the mid-nineteenth century the editor of the *Journal of Mental Science* believed he was in a position to declare that insanity was a brain disease. Pilgrim points out that this editorial pronouncement 'was made in the same year that the General Medical Bill passed through Parliament'. Under this 'the medical profession eventually gained a mandate from the State to define and manage certain forms of deviance as illness' (Pilgrim, 1992, p. 211). The 'responsible guardian of the lunatic', the psychiatrist, received state verification of his role. The conceptualization of madness in medical terms was socially validated by the state when it validated the medical profession as a whole.

Prior to the time at which the *Journal of Mental Science* declared insanity was disease, and the UK Parliament gave state support to the medical profession, there had been a period of struggle. To simplify, this took place between the physicians and the proponents of moral or psychological treatment, as Boyle

(1990, p. 20) calls it. If we look more closely at the struggle, the argument about the nature of madness, which one might expect to have had a scientific aspect, appears integrally entwined with the social changes.

The moral approach to madness originated in the UK with the work of Samuel Tuke at the York Retreat (cf. Porter, 1991, pp. 325–6) and in France with the work of Pinel at the Bicêtre and La Salpêtrière hospitals. Pinel, famously, took the shackles from the limbs of his patients. The views of the moral movement in the UK were associated with the reformist tendency of the first half of the nineteenth century. The reformers were seen by medicine as a threat to their existing control over lunacy and the asylums (see Scull, 1989, p. 137). The reformers tried to change the existing social organization of madness by introducing non-medical superintendence of asylums (*ibid.*, pp. 135–7) and making inspections of asylums by the civic authorities, in the form of magistrates, obligatory (*ibid.*, p. 140).

These attempts to change the social organization of madness did have some measure of success (*ibid.*, p. 150). Physician John Haslam was sacked from his post at the Bethlem Asylum after the report of an 1815 House of Commons investigation (Porter, 1988, particularly xxvi). But the advocates of the moral treatment and reform did not go unanswered. Scull lists more than 25 publications between 1815 and mid-century, which support the medical picture of insanity or recommend medical responses (Scull, 1989, p. 144n79). Without going into detail, the reformist tendency in the care of the mad had no long-term success. Politically, it finally failed in the House of Lords and in the face of effective medical lobbying (*ibid.*, pp. 140–2).

In terms of social organization:

> By the 1830s almost all the public mental hospitals had a resident medical director. Moreover, the magistrates' committees, which in several instances had been heavily involved in the day-to-day administration of asylums, increasingly left everything to the experts. . . . Similarly, in the private sector, the more reputable private institutions acquired either a medical proprietor or a full-time resident medical superintendent. Ibid. (p. 160)

Even Tuke's York retreat, from which moral treatment in the UK had originated, appointed a medical superintendent in 1838 (*ibid.*, p. 160 and n.151). A series of acts (Madhouse Act, 1828; Lunatics Act, 1845) and the gradual dominance of the medical profession among lunacy commissioners ensured that by mid-century, non-medics had either been forced out or subordinated everywhere (Scull, 1989, pp. 160–1). The moral treatment movement was a social failure: it lost out to the medics in the question of who was to have control over asylums and mad people.

How were matters decided?

Scull thinks that the social and political aspects were decisive in the revolution in madness, and quotes Friedson to that effect: 'the process determining the outcome was essentially political and social rather than technical in character, a process in which power and persuasive rhetoric were of greater importance than the objective character of the knowledge, training, and work' (p. 161; quoting Freidson, 1970, p. 79).

Scull does not rule out the idea that something of what was at stake in the struggle was to do with the 'objective character of the knowledge'. Quite what Scull intends by this phrase is not clear. But even supposing it refers to knowledge about an independently existing object of enquiry (mental illnesses of various kinds, for example) Scull still thinks that what determined the outcome of the struggle was the political and social.

This seems to be grist to a sceptic's mill. It appears to be another mark of pseudo-science related to the one already identified. We have already seen the claim that a pseudo-science creates its own objects out of the social, political, and ethical norms of the time. Additionally, perhaps, it typically gets its account of things accepted by social, political, and ethical means. Psychiatry in early nineteenth century UK succeeds as a (pseudo-)science by hitching itself to the political and social coat-tails of medicine generally. Medicine is an organized pressure group that has considerable clout in Parliament and outside it. The physicians of the time are able to influence the political process in such a way that not only do they gain state validation of their own exclusive rights to practice and self-regulation (in the 1858 Act) but they also win the political battle to take charge of the new state-sponsored system for the care of the lunatics.

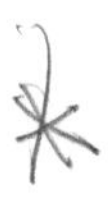

This is I believe what a sceptical account would look like of the events of the early nineteenth century regarding the nature of madness recounted by Scull and others. Certainly, it would have no room for any genuine medical scientific or conceptual discussion. However, there are other aspects of the same story to be revealed that potentially fit less easily within a sceptical view. Scull records more than the political and social manoeuvrings in the struggle between the reformists and the physicians. He recounts that there at least appeared to be a conceptual difference between them. The outcome of the social and political manoeuvrings was more than simply that physicians did as a matter of fact take charge of the mad. They also won a struggle to define the nature of madness.

At first sight this seems to go against the sceptic's view. True, the conceptual aspects of the struggle cannot be entirely separated from its social and political aspects. However, the direction of influence is plausibly from the conceptual to the social. We can identify a number of ways in which the conceptual position of the reformers tended to undermine their social and political credibility. For one thing, moral treatment did not identify a professional role for itself, while the physicians had a clear professional role. This was simply part and parcel of the reformers' denial that madness required special care (e.g. Scull, 1989, pp. 137ff). Moral treatment did not really present a clear organized alternative to medicine. Nor could moral treatment advance any rationale for why it should work; rather, it proceeded from and claimed to need no special explanatory model (see *ibid.*, pp. 153ff). Boyle describes it as pragmatic in its approach (1990, pp. 28, 29). Indeed, its boundaries with medicine were blurred to its disadvantage. It used some medical concepts in its terminology such as affliction, disease, and treatment (Scull, 1989, p. 138). This meant that the medical professionals could apparently smoothly integrate the concept of moral treatment within their armamentarium if and when they needed to, but the advocates of moral treatment could not absorb medicine in its entirety into theirs. The struggle was effectively ended when the medical profession offered to concede that moral treatment was indeed important. This concession left the doctors in effective possession of the entire field, for only they could offer what they said was the ideal regimen of both the medical and the moral treatments (*ibid.*, pp. 159–60).

Other aspects of the conceptual problems faced by the reformers were more purely abstract. There was an apparent inconsistency in their position. Their view of the mad was that they lacked self-control (cf. Porter, 1991, pp. 325–6). The medical profession successfully turned this notion that madness was a *moral* problem against the reformers. Doctors were able to point out that by Christian doctrine the mind or, what was the same thing, the soul, must be immortal and perfectible (Boyle, 1990, p. 27). The adherents of moral treatment could not effectively demur given their own adherence to the dominant Christian doctrine. But what was immortal could not be subject to deadly decay or disruption. So any disorder of the lunatic must be somatic, the result of changes in the brain through which the immortal mind was forced to operate. And the brain was part of the medical domain (Scull, 1989, pp. 155–7; Boyle, 1990, p. 27).

A sceptic would no doubt say that the argument between the sides about the nature of madness is more apparent than real, in so far as either or both wish to see madness as some form of illness. On the sceptic's account we would not be able to make sense of a disagreement wholly or partly couched in these terms. In so far as either side is committed to the illness story it is also committed to a metaphor. Neither the moral treaters nor the physicians could have produced anything but a metaphorical illness out of madness. Perhaps a sceptic would suggest that there is some alternative real reason for their acts (something we shall revisit with ADHD in the next chapter). They are really interested in extending their domain and hence their power. Whether or not insanity really is a moral or a medical matter is not the issue. The issue is whether a magistrate or a physician shall have the final say on what happens to mad people.

Moreover, as the alternatives have so far been described, they fit in with a sceptic's general analysis. We are left with the choice between saying that psychiatry is politics or ethics by an alternative (metaphorical) route, or that it is a genuine science that has independent objects and has a method of its own for sorting out its internal difficulties rather than relying on political and social power. However, I wish to dispute that this is the choice. Rather, I think we can admit the role of the human in creating the objects in which a science may be interested without admitting the idea that the human can create only political, or social or ethical objects. Metaphor can have a role in a genuine science in creating these objects.

6.4 Mental illness and the role of the social (2)

Finding a way in which metaphor can play a role in creating the objects of a genuine science relies upon keeping apart two ideas. These are the ideas that humans have a role in the creation of some of the objects of their own interest and investigation, and the idea that humans create the objects of their own investigation by means of and as a reflection of social, political, and ethical attitudes. I do not believe these two ideas have to become one.

None the less, it is not always as easy as all that to keep them apart. And there are reasons why this seems particularly difficult in the field in which we are principally interested. Scull's account of the development of the idea of mental illness in the late eighteenth and early nineteenth century seems at times to bring the two ideas under one roof. With psychiatry and mental illness there seems to be a case for saying that the creation of the objects of interest was after all the expression of certain social attitudes. These are the attitudes of late eighteenth century market capitalism. The case is that the very notion of mental illness is a reproduction of a social category produced by capitalism, and not, as presented by physicians at the time, a discoverable, objective state in nature. Scull's work provides a plausible basis for this case, though I do not wish to claim that he would make it himself, and am using his work only to illustrate how the case might be worked out in detail. I believe also that a sceptic such as Szasz would embrace it, at least in so far as he could restrict it to psychiatry.

However, as will soon appear, I do not think that the case can successfully be made out. I shall do my best to illustrate what would be entailed in showing that mental illness is a reproduction of a social category. That will be the task of the next subsection *Market capitalism and the idea of mental illness*. The subsequent subsection will demonstrate that seeking to show how scientific categories are actually social categories is part of the strong programme in the sociology of knowledge. In the two subsections following that I will lodge a general objection to the strong programme and then seek to show why in particular the attempt to show that mental illness is a reproduction of a social category must fail. The reason, to foreshadow the end-point of the discussion, is that the terms in which explanations of illness are couched (for instance those of causality) are not plausibly social terms. The metaphor of mental illness makes possible scientific forms of understanding and explanation.

Market capitalism and the idea of mental illness

Let us start by seeking to show what a case for saying that mental illness is a reproduction of a social category might look like.

Countering the claim that the growth of the nineteenth century asylum can be put down to the increasing urbanization of the late eighteenth century (Miller and Szasz, 1983 p. 272), Scull locates the cause in the earlier growth of market capitalism. His reasoning, not too distorted by abbreviation I hope, is this. A capitalist economy requires a labour market (Scull, 1989, p. 219). The force that was to drive people into this market was hunger and need (*ibid.*, pp. 219–20); this force could be viewed as a law of nature (*ibid.*, p. 220). The workhouse was a place into which those who were without work but still in hunger and need could be channelled. However, the supposed natural force driving them there did not distinguish the able-bodied from the non-able bodied; anyone who did not have a source of income might fall victim to it. The workhouses filled with all sorts.

A labour market can accept that some cannot work, and perhaps deserve support, but it cannot operate properly if this category is mixed up with people who are deliberately avoiding work, that is to say malingerers. The distinction of the able-bodied and able-minded from the non-able-bodied and non-able-minded is therefore required (*ibid.*, p. 219). The former must not be offered aid, but must seek work in the market (*ibid.*, p. 219). Once within the workhouses it was possible to identify some who seemed mentally either unwilling or unable to work by the house's rules (*ibid.*, p. 220). Particularly intractable were 'the acutely disturbed and refractory insane' (*ibid.*). By their actions they threatened the order and discipline of the whole workhouse leading to calls, both by authorities and fellow inmates, for their segregation (*ibid.*).

Scull's position is that segregation of this group of people was demanded within the capitalist system. We can go further perhaps and say the capitalist system created them, in the sense that it was in the context of the workhouse and its operations that their behaviour drew attention to them, whereas under the previous system they had not come up against such institutions or rules, and had been invisible. The position we are considering has to go further than this, however. It has to show that the idea that a person really is unable to earn his or her keep in the market is not an independent fact about any person, but is a vision of people possible only in terms of the market. It needs to show that the notion that some of those in the category of people who were unable to earn their keep were mentally ill is a fact of the same sort. This is what is needed to show what is claimed to be a natural or scientific category (that someone is ill) is a reproduction of a social category.

The argument would have to go something like this: it is only when people are thought about as potentially productive units in a market that the notion that some people fail to be such productive units can appear. And it is only when being productive is regarded as how people should be that some reason is needed to explain why they are not. The ideas come together. The group of people constituted by the 'acutely disturbed and refractory insane' were identifiable only in virtue of their being part of a larger group: those who fail, for one reason or another, to be productive. Their disturbance and refractoriness appears only against the expectation that they should act in a certain way, namely productively.

As Scull notes, certain forces, regarded as natural (hunger for example) were conceived of as driving people to the workhouses. The idea that there are such natural forces, it might be argued, is part and parcel of the market view of the world. So too might be the notion that those who ended up in the workhouses were either malingerers actually driven by this natural force but seeking to avoid its consequences, or in the grip of some other natural force that makes them unproductive (illness). In nature, we might say, there are no such categories. Medical science naturalizes what are in fact purely social distinctions. It does this by using naturalistic scientific category terms such as disease, diagnosis, and so forth.

As I have indicated, I think there are fundamental problems with this account. They lie in the use of the term reproduce. This glosses over differences between the descriptions of the social and natural worlds that would otherwise undermine the idea that one could reproduce the one in the other. However, supposing the account could overcome this, it appears to lend support to a sceptic. Actually, or so it appears to show, there is nothing in nature that could lead us to the distinction of the able and non-able minded among people. Likewise a sceptic such as Szasz claims there is no objective distinction between health and ill-health, which will correlate with disvalued behaviours. We make the distinction of able and non-able-minded people by means of our social values (e.g. productivity), which is to say in the light of our social beliefs. Market capitalism creates this distinction. We then project it into nature. And then we purport to have found it there. We do this when we announce that there are causal connections between the brain or the genes and schizophrenia. But in fact, psychiatric medicine can be seen to be based not upon the reality of such a distinction in nature, biology, or anatomy, but upon the market capitalist's social exclusion of the unproductive. Mental illness is the apparent means of making the distinction; but the distinction itself is social. Mental illness is not a feature of the natural world around us, though psychiatrists speak as if it were. It is actually a feature of the capitalist view of society.[2] There is no room in this account for a metaphor that creates the object of a genuine scientific study.

As can be seen the two ideas that I was earlier trying hard to keep apart have here apparently been forced together. These ideas are that humans may have a part in creating the objects of their own study, and the idea that humans create some things out of social materials. And where these ideas come together, if mental illness is a metaphor, the role of the human imagination in the creation of the objects of science turns out to be the projection of a social, political, and ethical attitude on to nature. The example of mental illness and psychiatry in the nineteenth century seems to be a case in point. Psychiatry has turned out to be market capitalism by other means. And this fits in with a sceptic's general analysis and seems to lead us towards his or her conclusion: psychiatry is a pseudo-science.

However, it would be a mite too hasty simply to accept what I have suggested would be the sceptical gloss on this. There are two reasons for this. First, because a far more general analysis very like the one I have just been giving of psychiatry is to be found within the philosophy of science, where it is given as an account of all science. The foregoing discussion has been shadowing the strong programme in the sociology of knowledge. Indeed, my discussion has quite deliberately tried to shadow this programme. It is an important discussion for us to consider. It takes an analysis of the kind we have just been giving of psychiatry, and denies that this is the mark of something unusual among the sciences, or the mark of a pseudo-science. It is in fact, according to the strong programme in the sociology of knowledge, the correct account of anything that takes the name of science. In that sense the strong programme furnishes us with a possible source of a response to the sceptic. The sceptic wants to distinguish psychiatry from medicine as a pseudo-science, but this is a recourse the strong programme denies.

The second reason for doubting the sceptical gloss on the account of psychiatric categories given in this subsection is this: it is far from clear that the case that mental illness is a reproduction of a social category has successfully been made out.

We may deal with each of these points in turn, starting in the next subsection with a brief presentation of the strong programme, and moving in subsequent subsection to a critique of this.

The strong programme in the sociology of knowledge

The strong programme in the sociology of knowledge starts from the idea that knowledge and the categories and classifications of things are closely related. This is a claim I have broadly accepted. I have supposed that the notion of mental illness is such a category closely related to the possibility of knowledge in psychiatry: 'All systems of knowledge . . . are constituted by the divisions that are drawn between kinds or sorts of thing. Distinguishing like from unlike; deciding what is to count as likeness or unlikeness; balancing the consequences of those decisions; this is how our understanding becomes an orderly affair.' (Bloor, 1982, p. 267).

What marks the strong programme out, and what we will later question, is its claim that the propositions of scientific knowledge 'in themselves embody social factors' (Knorr-Cetina, 1983, p. 116, quoted by Chalmers, 1990, p. 91). To put this claim in another way: human knowledge cannot be expressed without recourse to categories of things, and the categories of things have an irreducibly social content.

David Bloor, one the strong programme's proponents, gives a specification of this general position which is of particular interest to us. He uses a phrase of Durkheim's: The classification of things reproduces the classification of men (Bloor, 1982, p. 267; Durkheim and Mauss, 1903, p. 11). That is to say things around us are classified into the same sorts of classes we classify people. Our classifications of people produce a 'pattern of social inclusions and exclusions' (Bloor, 1982, p. 267). Social inclusions and exclusions are things like class, conformity, productivity, and other normative features based upon differing values and attitudes. Our categories of things (animals, trees, physical and mental illness, atomic and subatomic particles) are supposed to reproduce these.

By the lights of the strong programme, if the phrase madness is illness is a proposition of scientific knowledge it will embody social inclusions and exclusions. These will in turn be produced by attitudes, beliefs, values, or whatever. Because scientific knowledge is the embodiment of the social in this way, it is constituted by historically mutable and diverse cultures in their own image. This account of science carries the social into the very heart of science, that is into the very propositions science regards as stating what we know, for instance, as we will discuss shortly, into notions such as those to be found in Newtonian physics.

It is of course unwise altogether to deny the role of the social in science. We can study how some research programmes come to be well funded and others fail to get going for lack of support. However, the strong programme is not content with showing how social forces can influence funding and publication of research, and other elements of the social success of scientists and their enterprises. Showing this kind and level of social involvement in science comprises the weak programme in the sociology of knowledge. The weak programme would be concerned with the social and political manoeuvrings by which nineteenth century doctors achieved their goal of control over the mad. It was these aspects we were principally interested in in Section 3 of this chapter. The weak programme would content itself with revealing these and their role in the development of psychiatry as a social institution. But it would stop short of showing that a claim such as 'insanity is a disease of the brain' is itself dependent upon social values.

Objections to the strong programme can consist in showing that what is true about it is what is true about the weak programme, though this truth is not philosophically or scientifically all that interesting. We shall shortly be asking general questions about the validity of the strong programme. For now my question shall be: could the strong programme apply to psychiatry; specifically, did the account of the role of capitalism in the development of the notion of mental illness, given in the previous subsection, establish a case consistent with the strong programme?

The strong programme would certainly have to apply to psychiatry in the eyes of those who take the position of the strong programme. This is because the theses of the strong programme are entirely general. All putative scientific knowledge is supposed to fall under them, including that of natural sciences, the medical sciences, the social sciences, and philosophy (cf. Bloor, 1976, p. 65). In fact, the proponents of the strong programme do not really recognize the distinction between social and natural sciences so far as the nature of their knowledge is concerned. And nor do they recognize the distinction identified earlier between what are usually called pseudo-sciences and genuine sciences. This is not surprising. According to the strong programme, all sciences, and not merely those that are sometimes called metaphorical or pseudo-sciences, create their objects by creating the categories of things. This makes the strong programme useless for a sceptic's purposes.

Consistent with this, the proponents of the strong programme when applied in individual cases have been particularly keen to show how the hardest of hard science reveals social factors. The strong programme aims to identify the actual sources of the irreducible social component in specific examples of what is or has been said to be known by science (Bloor, 1976, pp. 26–8). Bloor on different occasions looks at the work of Newton (Bloor, 1982) and the propositions of mathematics (Bloor, 1976).

What Bloor says about Newton is particularly worth noting in the light of our purposes. Newton's view of the physical world is like Descartes': that it is mechanistic. His status as a scientist is exalted, so he makes a particularly prized target. Bloor holds up Newton's theories as examples of the way in which social and political views shape and give content to scientific knowledge in the most fundamental science. Newton's fundamental corpuscular notions about the physical world are said to reproduce his view of the atomistic yet law governed nature of society. The fundamental particles (atoms), of which Newton thought the physical world is ultimately constituted, are supposed to be unable to move themselves, and to be subject to control only by forces outside them. This, it is claimed, reproduces Newton's political and social views. He was a member of a social group, led by Boyle, opposed to the idea that each individual can find and follow his or her own religious and moral light. Boyle and Newton did not believe individuals should, in this sense, be self-moving. They believed that individuals are properly subject to the external authority of the established church. The individual members of society are the atoms of Newton's political philosophy. His atomist mechanist political philosophy was expressed in his atomist mechanist physics. That is to say, his theories reproduce his vision of society (Bloor, 1982; see also Chalmers, 1990, pp. 104–12).

This seems straightforward on the surface, but a problem arises about the exact meaning of the claim that the classification of things *reproduces* the classification of people, as Bloor acknowledges (Bloor, 1982, p. 269). The notion of reproducing needs to be specified. A relation of reproduction can be one of copying: in this sense, a photographic reproduction of *The Haywain* is a copy of the original. But this sense of copy cannot be what Bloor wants. The copy of *The Haywain* is a copy in virtue of having the same colours and shades of colour arranged more or less exactly as in the original. But the atoms, forces, and laws in Newton's physics are nothing like the atoms, forces, and laws in his politics. In another use of the term reproduce, we may reproduce and predict the action of water in a mathematical model. But again, this seems the wrong idea for Bloor's purposes. Newton may be modelling his physical theories on his social beliefs, but he is presumably not attempting to use his corpuscles to work out what will happen to people, or *vice versa*.

In answer to his own question about what reproduce means Bloor uses Mary Douglas's words: 'Apprehending a general pattern of what is right and necessary in social relations is the basis of society: this apprehension generated whatever a priori or set of necessary causes is going to be found in nature.' (Douglas, 1975, p. 281 n38; Bloor, 1982, p. 283).

The claim is we project upon the natural world a series of a prioris or necessities. These are not actually in the natural world, and are not actually a priori or necessary, in the sense of being forced upon us by the natural world. Newton thought that individuals should not be self-moving, but should bow to higher authority in society. He took the notion of non-self-moving and used it in the sphere of physics. There it turns into what seems to be a description of how things are, and perhaps how they must be.

A parallel example can be described in such a way as to illustrate Douglas'/Bloor's point. In some views *in vitro* fertilization (IVF) is said to be unnatural as it interferes with the unity of the natural process of human reproduction. But those who support IVF often argue that we now know that natural human reproduction is actually a series of events connected only by contingency, and have no natural unity. Which of these two views of nature is right? Nature does not tell us herself; she is the object of the disagreement. Rather, as Bloor says, she is 'put to social use' (Bloor, 1982, p. 283). 'Certain [so-called natural] laws are protected and rendered stable because of their assumed utility for purposes of justification, legitimation and social persuasion' (*ibid.*). No doubt if the anti-IVF lobby dominated, the idea that human procreation presents us with a natural unity would appear entirely obvious, and would guide our attitude to IVF. However, from the view of the strong programme, whichever version of nature we thought true, our attitude to IVF, and other such interventions, would actually be being reproduced (see Pickering, 1996).

Applied to our earlier example of Newton, the atomist political beliefs about how individuals should be are projected upon nature where they become a belief about how atoms behave, and get given the status of a law of nature.

Objections to the strong programme

The strong programme in the sociology of knowledge is a radical programme, at least in one important sense. One thing it does is to take the sceptical criticism of psychiatry we have been considering and turn it on its head. In the eyes of the strong programme if psychiatry is in effect the imposition of social and ethical views through the purported objectivity of science, then it is no more and no less a science than physical medicine, Newtonian or post-Newtonian physics, and mathematics. All these purport to have found or be investigating certain laws (of nature or of number) but in reality they are reproducing among numbers and within nature the social attitudes of the physicists and mathematicians. The strong programme is not conducive to sceptical ideas about psychiatry—it is not radical in that sense. But it is radical in the sense that it denies the contrast between genuine objective science based upon the laws of anatomy (physical medicine) and pseudo or metaphorical science based on human beliefs (psychiatry).

Not surprisingly such a radical programme has its opponents. One thing they object to is the way in which science and pseudo-science are run together. They seek to show that science has characteristic resources by which it divides what can be called scientific knowledge from mere speculation or wishful thinking. Alan Chalmers quarrels with the example of Newton Bloor uses. Chalmers argues that we can distinguish between what was genuine science in Newton's theories and what was pseudo-science. If we look into history we can in fact see this distinction being demonstrated. Parts of Newton's theories have been confirmed by later observation and experiment, in particular his laws of motion. But other parts of his theories have not received confirmation, and have in fact been abandoned. Clerk Maxwell's is a good example here: 'Clerk Maxwell departed radically from the fundamental particle assumption when he utilized Newtonian mechanics to develop his electromagnetic field theory, in which localized phenomena are understood in terms of the mechanics of a continuous, all-pervasive material medium . . . .' (Chalmers, 1990, p. 111). This is intended to serve as a refutation of Bloor's claim that scientific knowledge is determined by the social views of scientists. Though a scientist may come up with his ideas from resources that include his or her social and ethical attitudes, there is still an independent way of formulating and judging the worth of these ideas in scientific terms. When this independent mode of scientific judgement is applied to Newton's theories, parts of them are dropped. In particular, the corpuscular theory (the fundamental particle assumption), according to Chalmers, was found wanting and was abandoned. And this is the part of Newton's theory that Bloor's account concentrates upon.

Chalmers' general case is that the acceptance of some aspect of a theory for social or other non-scientific reasons is in principle different from its acceptance for scientific reasons. That is to say, Chalmers broadly accepts the distinction between what are known as the context of discovery and the context of justification (though he insists on some qualifications and clarifications of this distinction). The context of discovery, it is usually held, can be anything you like. Newton's corpuscular theories can be put down to his religious, social, and ethical views. But they could, Chalmers holds, have been justified on scientific grounds. The motions of the corpuscles relative to absolute space might have become detectable and their counting might have become possible (Chalmers, 1990, p. 111). So, 'while certain assumptions had their origins in seventeenth-century social changes and social theory, they only received an adequate scientific interpretation and justification centuries later. We would have a situation similar to the one which traces some of Darwin's innovations to the writings of Malthus and the social situation that inspired them.' (*Ibid.*).

But when it comes to formulating and testing a scientist's ideas, science has its own set of methods and resources. It uses these to interpret the scientist's claim, putting it into a testable form, and then to apply experiment and/or observation to it. Until these tests are applied, and perhaps even afterwards, a theory may hold sway for social or political reasons. However, as Chalmers points out, politically correct science turns out often to be bad science. The Russian biologist Lysenko was not a good scientist despite his endorsement by the dominant Soviet regime (Chalmers, 1990, p. 82). Which is to say, the arbiter of scientific assertions is not the Party, the ballot box, or the *coup d'état*. Scientists may be motivated by desire for personal gain, by political ideology, by fear, or even by moral considerations. But when, in the face of the threats of the Inquisitors, Galileo recanted his view that the solar system was heliocentric, and then said under his breath that it was really, he was not contradicting himself. He was making a political statement, and then a scientific statement. They answer to different authorities.

I do not find either Chalmer's position or that of Bloor entirely satisfactory in the particular case of psychiatry. The role of evidence for scientifically formulated propositions seems less clear in the case of psychiatry than Chalmer's position would require.

Mental illness and the strong programme

The claim of the editor of the *Journal of Mental Science* was that insanity was a brain disease. This claim was made in 1858. William Cullen in the previous century made the claim that a problem of the nerves generally (neurosis) was the explanation of a good deal of madness. An obvious test for mental illness conceived as a brain disease would be the finding of the brain lesions Victorian alienists claimed were there. So, even if we accept that the very idea of mental incapacity is the creation of the ideology of market capitalism reproduced as if it were a natural aspect of the physical world, we can still ask for scientific proof of this claim. This means giving it a testable formulation and testing it.

In reality things were rather different. No such lesions were identifiable at the time, and this was well known. The failure to find the lesions was explained by nineteenth century physicians, according to Scull. They argued that instruments of the day were too crude to detect the structural lesions in the brain; and that they developed grossly enough to be seen only in the later stages of disease (when it was claimed lesions could be found) but not in the early stages (Scull, 1989, p. 157; Boyle, 1990, p. 27). This hardly explains the continuing success of the physical medical explanation in the face of a further century of failures to find brain lesions. Indeed, this failure was compounded by the collapse, in the period after 1845 or so, of the pretensions of the medicalized asylums to provide a cure (Scull, 1989, p. 235; see also Boyle, 1990, p. 34). What can explain this continuing classificatory success in the face of an evident lack of success finding what would appear to be scientific or therapeutic support for it?

Those who believe that psychiatry is a genuine science in the sense allowed by the sceptic may have some difficulties explaining this. The role of evidence in scientific rationality is usually taken to be clear. It can be seen as the point at which human theories about what the world should do come up against what it actually does. It represents the point at which reality constrains theory. Here, however, we have the acceptance of the notion of mental illness despite the substantial absence of evidence. This tells against the idea that science is entirely a self-contained, self-verifying thing. Somehow, despite the apparent evidential situation, psychiatry carried on as if it was a law of nature that madness was caused by brain lesions.

This fits in well with Bloor's position. He argues that the role of evidence in particular cases is not given but depends on social factors (Bloor, 1976). Of this, the nineteenth century development of the science of psychiatry seems to be a good example, as Scull suggests. The lack of evidence did not lead then nor has it led since to the rejection of psychiatry or mental illness or to specific diagnoses within psychiatry, though Boyle believes it should have in the case of schizophrenia (see 1990, pp. 6, 72–3). Psychiatry has traded virtually throughout on the idea that in due course the physical bases of mental illnesses will be revealed (Boyle, 1990, p. 168). The relation of the evidential situation to the claims of psychiatry can be determined when we take into account non-scientific factors. Bloor of course makes this a general claim about all science. I wish only to note that it seems at first sight to fit the case of psychiatry.

Perhaps Chalmers would reply that just because, as a matter of historical fact, a claim is held despite the complete lack of evidence for it, does not show that there is not a way in which the claim could be tested scientifically. Here I think Chalmers is right. And Bloor appears to supply a good illustration in the case of Lord Kelvin's objections to the theory of evolution for Chalmers' claim against his own (see 1976, p. 4). Lord Kelvin's arguments against evolution were rejected by nineteenth century geologists and biologists even though they could not see what was wrong with them. Kelvin argued that the sun could be only so many years old or it would have burned out, and that given this there was not sufficient time for evolution to have taken place. The gradual accumulation of the fossil record finally persuaded scientists that Kelvin's objections were implausible, but nothing was found that contradicted his reasoning or assumptions. Lord Kelvin's position was simply ignored. Bloor records, however, that in the twentieth century the discovery that the sun had nuclear sources of energy showed that Kelvin's objections were based on a physical mistake (about the nature of processes within the sun). But, this latter point, that Kelvin's physical theories were mistaken seems to be exactly what Chalmers wants, for surely this is a matter of testing by later *science*. Bloor's own example illustrates the distinction Chalmers makes use of against him.

However, there is a sting in the tail for psychiatry. The problem is to show that science really can decide the acceptability of claims such as insanity is brain disease altogether on its own terms. Discovering brain lesions might indeed have fulfilled the criterion set by nineteenth century medicine. However, the criterion even if met falls short of determining the matter, as the earlier discussion (in Chapter 2) of alcoholism, ADHD, and schizophrenia suggested. The presence of correlating brain lesions to the behavioural patterns of the alcoholic shows nothing without a further presumption of the right kind of relation between them. The right kind of relation would appear to be causal in nature. However, whether we view the relation as causal or as an occasion of temptation is itself internally related to whether we think alcoholism is an illness or not. The same goes for idea that the body is a machine (Chapter 5). There can be no evidence for such claims independent of accepting them (this is a point we will explore further in Chapter 8). The strong view of the mistake in likeness arguments supports the doubts raised here about the capacity of evidence to test such claims as madness is a brain disease.

Chalmers' method for showing that the strong programme in the sociology of knowledge must fail in physics does not transfer to the situation with psychiatry and mental illness in the nineteenth century in the UK in a straightforward fashion. Nor could it. Chalmers' attack on Bloor's analysis is based upon the idea that science has justificatory means at its disposal to test the hypotheses of scientists. Science formulates knowledge claims in testable ways and can appeal to observation and evidence. However, in the case of schizophrenia, alcoholism, ADHD, depression, and other so-called mental illnesses the existence of much of the evidence in question is tied to beliefs about their medical status. The tests in question are still those of observation and experiment, but we can see that the material with which these operate—the evidence itself—has its character predetermined. Those who sought correlating brain lesions in the nineteenth century and those who seek correlating brain lesions in the twentieth century both presume that the correlating lesions stand in a causal relationship with the behaviours in question. But whether they do is a further question the identification of the correlations cannot itself answer.

So this may all turn out to be grist to a sceptic's mill, if Chalmers is right about indubitably genuine sciences, such as physics. Newton's theories have been formulated and tested by physicists, and some of them found wanting, while others have survived. But this analysis may not work in the case of psychiatry. If so, that seems to be all the worse for psychiatry as a genuine science, and all the better for the sceptic. Moreover, it seems to be conformable to my account of the likeness argument. The illness-like features by which we might have judged the claim (say) that schizophrenia is an illness, appear only in the light of the idea that (say) schizophrenia is an illness. Boyle says: 'It might . . . reasonably be argued that the *language*, or the *idea*, of behaviour as illness and of 'schizophrenia' as a particular and serious form of illness is important in maintaining the impression of similarity between psychiatry and the various medical specialties, in the absence of some important actual similarities in their activities.' (1990, p. 179).

My position seems in danger of collapsing into one of scepticism.

However, although, as I have suggested, the existence and nature of the so-called evidence that schizophrenia or alcoholism are illnesses are predetermined by the views of the scientists that they are illnesses, the nature of the physical (or functional) connection that is said to exist is not social. Medical scientists of the nineteenth century, and no doubt medical scientists today seek causal connections. Furthermore, they seek these connections among the biological, structural, and functional aspects of the human being. The causal nature of these connections, and the physical or functional nature of the fabric or medium in which they are said to be found, means that they are not social connections. Certainly, this is what a sceptic like Szasz holds about the differences between the social and the medical. And it is a view I hold to some degree too: The social arena is one that is described to some degree in terms other than those in which a psychiatrist describes her arena. The notion of behaviour is a descriptive resource of the social scientist, or the historian perhaps, in looking at various human phenomena. It cannot, or so a sceptic would say, be mixed up with the descriptive resources of psychiatry.

However, this is not to deny psychiatry its own descriptive resources, and its own kind of interest. We find ourselves making a point that we earlier noticed Szasz himself making. That is that the nature of our interest in some things is not decided by those things, rather, what sort of thing we think those things are reveals the nature of our interest. This is certainly out of tune with much else of what Szasz says and with his dominant scepticism. It does not entail denying the existence of mental illness, for example. None the less it strikes me as the right note to strike. The psychiatrist takes a causal interest in the nature of schizophrenia, and reveals this in what she says about the relation of the genes or the brain or the mind to the condition called schizophrenia. She describes it in ways internally related to this kind of interest. The sceptic takes a non-medical interest, and reveals this in what he or she says about schizophrenia being a behaviour. So, though the psychiatrist to some degree creates the connections between brain, or mind functions, and the symptoms of mental illness, it is important that it is in these terms that she works. These are the terms that psychiatry has developed over the historical period of its existence; and it is in the light of these ideas that psychiatry constructs its objects.

The same point can be made about Bloor's attempts to show that the content of philosophical theories and of scientific theories is a reproduction of social, political, and religious ideology. One example of this reproduction is the following: 'The antithesis of individualistic democracy and collectivist, paternalist authoritarianism is apparent in [Popper's and Kuhn's] theories of knowledge. Popper's theory is anti-authoritarian and atomistic; Kuhn's is holistic and authoritarian.' (Bloor, 1976, p. 65).

This is supposed to help persuade us that their philosophical theories reproduce their creators' social and political standpoints. Bloor achieves this persuasive effect by describing Popper's and Kuhn's theories in terms friendly to his claim. We are asked to accept that a theory of knowledge such as Popper's, which claims that theories can only be falsified and never be verified, is anti-authoritarian in the same sense as individualistic democracy is anti-authoritarian. However, we may want to question whether the authority of a theory in science and the authority of a government in political and social life are really points of analogy (as Bloor simply assumes). Likewise, we may doubt if a person who bows to the authority of the Church in religious matters is doing what an atom does when it is reacting to the forces of the physical world. Following Tirrell, we may perceive here a figurative likeness or reproduction. That is to say Bloor's own theory may then rely upon a series of metaphorical reproductions. This is not a refutation, to my mind, of Bloor's theory; for me this is evidence that he is using his imagination. It does, however, suggest that theory does not necessarily arise from the sifting of independent empirical evidence, but instead relies upon and reveals a certain way of thinking of that evidence.

So the idea that the social is *reproduced* in the fabric of the science of psychiatry has to be slightly amended, or the notion of reproduction has to be understood in a particular way. Chalmers is right to say that science can formulate things in its own terms. Psychiatrists formulate their account of schizophrenia, or alcoholism, in causal, physical, and functional terms. These terms are distinct from the terms in which we generally formulate an account of human behaviour. Unless we think of behaviour in the same set of terms, then we are able to make this distinction. And like many distinctions we make, it is one we carry through into the way we look at things around us. It is not, *pace* Szasz, a merely linguistic or verbal distinction: it is a classificatory distinction. We can, of course, think of behaviour in such causal terms, or of science in social terms. These are themselves possible recategorizations represented by metaphors.

If this is correct, then we have reason to think that we can keep apart the two ideas that sceptics such as Szasz (in his critique of psychiatry) and the proponents of the strong programme in the sociology of knowledge (in their account of science in general) run together. The terms in which psychiatry speaks of schizophrenia, depression, anxiety, and so on are not themselves social terms—the terms that would apply to behaviours. They represent a distinct way of looking at the phenomena associated with certain human conditions. Because they are not social terms themselves, they cannot necessarily in a simple sense reproduce the social values and ideas of the scientists in what is said to be natural or physical or functional.

At the same time, Chalmers' claim that such basic assumptions can be formulated and tested in scientific terms is now subject to some doubt. As the strong view of the mistake in likeness arguments suggests, the description of alcoholism and schizophrenia in non-social terms reflects a metaphor, a recategorization. It does not necessarily reflect a move either based upon or subject to evidential testing. Chalmers fails to leave room for the imaginative creation of such evidence though the recategorizing of metaphor. Of this creation of evidence we shall have much more to say in Chapter 8.

Conclusions

The different possible ways of thinking of the phenomena around us are marked out in part by our categories, classifications, and kinds. These categories are made up of the religious, social, moral, and political and of the scientific, mechanical, and causal. We take the kinds of interests represented by these categories in such matters as madness, and make it in the image of those interests. In the case of psychiatry, what makes it a scientific endeavour and what makes mental illness an object of that endeavour, is that psychiatry makes mental illness in non-social categories.

This position is, I believe, consistent with what is right in the strong programme in the sociology of knowledge. That is to say, it is consistent with what that programme can plausibly show, if not consistent with what it actually claims. It claims to show that political, economic, moral ideas are reproduced in scientific and other disciplines (including philosophy). But when we look carefully at the nature of this reproduction we see that it does not get as far as breaking down the distinction between the scientific and the social. There continues to be a case for a dualism. This dualism is perhaps less between the product of nature and the product of the social (the dualism of Latour's modern), and more between scientific resources and materials and social resources and materials. I would base my claim not to be a sceptic on the foundation of a dualism of this sort.

So, in the end, as I understand it, the strong programme is not a threat to my position. I can happily concur with what it can plausibly claim about the role of the social, while not being logically committed to anything more sceptical.

However, my appeal to the distinction between the scientific and natural (on the one hand) and the social on the other can be subjected to a sceptical challenge from another quarter. This challenge goes under the name of social constructionism. The sort of rhetoric that can be found in sceptical social constructionist approaches to mental illness echoes my own rhetoric uncomfortably. I have talked a good deal about mental illness being the creation of people, or of society. My central claim for metaphor tries to suggest how this creation might proceed. But it is a standard claim of the social constructionist that things that seemed to be produced by nature are after all produced by humans. This leads to the question: has the argument of this book in effect committed me to a sceptical social constructionist position?

I shall look at this question in the next chapter in the context of a specific issue: the illness status of ADHD. A strong case has been made that ADHD is a social construction and that this is a cause for scepticism about its status as a psychiatric diagnosis. I shall want to try to show how my case differs from this sceptical social constructionist one and defend the idea that ADHD is a metaphor.

Endnotes

1 It might be said that one thing the new set of descriptive terms does is to suggest the previous way of speaking or thinking of the area in question was metaphorical. Once the heliocentric view of the solar system had triumphed, the way the old geocentric view arose from metaphors such as 'man is the centre of universe' became clearer, though one might also say that 'man is the centre of the universe' became metaphorical once the earth had been physically marginalized. I owe this point to Peter Marshall (personal communication). Abrams (1953, p. 31) suggests that 'Even the traditional language of the natural sciences cannot claim to be totally literal, although its key terms often are not recognized to be metaphors until, in the course of time, the general adoption of a new analogy yields perspective into the nature of the old'.

2 For a claim plausibly of a similar kind, see Svensson (1990, p. 131). Taking his notion of ideology to cover such things as the market capitalist view of the world, he says 'Ideology designates a certain view, or interpretation, of certain phenomena that is associated with and serves, certain specifiable interests. . . . The ideological function of a conceptual model would then consist in its application to certain phenomena having the result that those phenomena were viewed or interpreted or categorized in a way that served certain interests (and perhaps thereby disrupted certain other interests).'

7 Attention deficit hyperactivity disorder, social construction, and metaphor

Physicians, by natural bent and by training, as well as by self-interest, are motivated to believe that they are dealing with biological disorders suitable for medical treatment.

Breggin (1998, p. 179)

7.1 Introduction

In this chapter I shall apply some of my thinking to ADHD. This means setting out an argument for the claim that the behaviours that are referred to by the term ADHD are made into an illness by metaphor. That is to say ADHD represents their being imaginatively categorized as illness, and so ADHD is a human creation in the sense developed in the last chapter. However, I shall resist the argument that its being a creation of the human imagination implies that ADHD is merely a social construct that cannot play any role in a genuine science.

In the previous chapter I also opposed a sceptical approach to mental illness modelled upon the strong programme in the sociology of knowledge. Social constructionism is not a programme, but is certainly a style of argument. (Social constructionism is the term Ian Hacking has suggested is used for the style I shall be describing in what follows. Sometimes, the term cultural is substituted for social; Latour has dropped the term 'social' altogether. In other areas, something similar seems to go under rather different names, e.g. constructivism in mathematics. See Hacking, 1999, pp. 47ff.) This style of argument can be seen as seeking to unmask ADHD by showing that it is an idea which has a social function. (I shall consider the notion of unmasking in more detail in Section 2 below.) This, from the sceptical social constructionist's position, can be taken to be tantamount to the conclusion that it is not real. I shall interpret this as meaning that it does not have an existence of the kind it is supposed to have, that is to say the kind of existence implicit in the medical approach.

I said at the close of the previous chapter that I need to show how my ideas differ from the social constructionist's. But I also commented that this presents a challenge because there are similarities. I have suggested previously that the creation of mental illness through metaphor is a historical event. The historical approach is certainly to be found in social constructionism. However, though my focus on history is consistent with the social constructionist approach, contrary to the claims of social constructionists I shall suggest ADHD itself is not constructed from the material of historical narratives, but out of medical materials. And this is why I do not hold that the emergence through metaphor of ADHD is reason for a sceptical conclusion about its illness status. These medical materials are distinct from the social (historical) materials that, the social constructionist would try to suggest, is what ADHD is actually made of.

However, this claim—that ADHD is constructed from medical materials—may also seem to be close to one made by social constructionists. For example the piece of rhetoric that heads this chapter, and this (also from Breggin): '. . . since the inception of psychiatry, psychiatrists as medical doctors have always claimed that everything they happen to be treating is biological and genetic. The claims, in other words, are nothing new. They are not scientifically based. They are inherent in the medical viewpoint.' (p. 173).

Breggin's claim that ADHD exists only in the light of the psychiatrists' particular interests and viewpoints is quite similar, I think, to my claim that mental illness is created from scientific materials: for it is likely that the constructors are psychiatrists (or more broadly, medical scientists). However, I shall be chiefly interested in a slightly broader version of the claim, which aims to show that ADHD exists only relative to social forces of some description. On this broader claim, it may be that ADHD reflects a wider social settlement rather than the interests of a specific group. None the less, I think my position still seems very close to that of a sceptical social constructionism.

Why attention deficit hyperactivity disorder?

ADHD is good contemporary example to test my ideas on because there is a large and vigorous literature already established concerning its illness status. Moreover, this literature is frequently divided over the question of social construction. Introducing a *British Journal of Psychiatry* discussion of ADHD 'Is ADHD best understood as a cultural construct?' Cannon, McKenzie and Sims comment: 'Fundamental to the discussion are questions about whether the diagnosis of ADHD actually holds water and what it is that psychiatrists are trying to treat. Are differences in the rate of ADHD a reflection of changes in its incidence or in society's tolerance for behaviour that does not conform?' (Timimi and Taylor, 2004, p. 8).

Here Cannon *et al.* set out radical questions such as the ones we have been interested in throughout the book, and put them in social constructionist terms. For example they ask how we are to explain differences from place to place and time to time in the amount of ADHD that is diagnosed. Do these differences reflect the fact that ADHD is more common in some places than in others? Or do they reflect variations in tolerance of the non-conformist behaviour ADHD labels? The radical question, whether ADHD is a diagnosis that 'holds water', is glossed as the question whether ADHD is what it claims to be (an illness) or exists only as a reflection of attitudes in society (a social construction).

Illina Singh, who inclines to a social constructionist approach to ADHD, identifies a similar sort of choice. She notes that 'environmental explanations' and 'the biological perspective' mark the extremes of a 'sharply polarized debate about the true causes of symptomatic behaviors and the legitimacy of diagnosis and treatment' (2002, p. 578). On one side of this divide (the biological side, as Singh calls it) it is said that ADHD is a legitimate diagnosis, that ADHD is a disease or illness entity (expressed in developmental deficits), that there is significant evidence for the claim that it is caused by brain malfunctioning, in turn caused by localized abnormalities in the brain. This side looks to drugs—in particular stimulants such as Ritalin—to deal with the problem. It also claims that ADHD shows up not only in children but in adults as well in ways that match the more advanced developmental stages of adults compared with children. (For example, the problems of adult ADHD will not lie in attending in class, but in attending in workplace meetings or at office computer stations.) It tends to be a somewhat expansionist approach (cf. Conrad and Potter, 2000).

On the other side of the divide (what Singh calls the environmental side) it is held that ADHD is a social or cultural construction (a reflection of social attitudes towards non-conformity, as Cannon *et al.* put it). It is held that the group of those said to have ADHD are in fact created by having the so-called illness attributed to them (by others or sometimes by the 'sufferers' themselves) on the basis of their unwanted and disvalued behaviours. This side holds that the so-called evidence of brain causality is misleading—that just because some brain states are supposedly correlated to the unwanted or disvalued behaviours does not prove that the behaviours have a biological origin. It holds that the use of drugs, far from being a cure for the problem represents a form of social control—children are being drugged for the convenience of harassed or incompetent parents, teachers, and social workers, or at least for the ease of society in general that would rather blame the children than blame itself. The extension of ADHD to adults—sometimes by self-attribution—is perceived as a parallel evasion of responsibility. ADHD is useful as a target of blame: it is useful for adults who have failed and who are looking for a quick fix for their lives rather than asking more fundamentally what might be wrong with the life choices they have made; and it is useful for society that would rather not ask questions about the kinds of choice of work and opportunities for a fulfilling life it imposes on its adult population.

The debate from which I have abstracted these two mutually exclusive positions is not actually quite so neatly divided as this description of the two sides would suggest. Many individual writers sit on the fence. But even where individual writers (there are many of them) do not fall simply into one camp or the other, they often see the issues in terms of the 'medical' versus 'social constructionist' debate (cf. Fukuyama, Elliott, Diller). Elliott, for example, who does not wholly reject the idea of ADHD, says that 'the real question is whether the diagnosis itself is a way of medicalising inattention and rowdiness' (2003, p. 251).

If these are really the choices we have, then my position seems to be forced into the social constructionist camp. But my comment on this debate is that it is misconceived. This appears in its presuppositions about what the alternatives actually are. These alternatives reflect the purist dualism of conceptual frameworks Latour attributes to the moderns and which we have noted previously. On the one hand, there are things that arise from nature: these are the objects of scientific investigation, according to the modern. Then there are other objects that are created by society—by human hand. In line with this dichotomy, those on both sides of this particular debate suppose that ADHD is either a social product (in which case it has no reality) or is a feature of the natural world (in which case it is real after all).

But perhaps ADHD is not a feature of the natural world, and yet is not a social product either. This, broadly speaking, is the conclusion I shall put forward. ADHD is the product of human imagination, but it is conceptualized in terms of relationships among the natural materials of the world. My answer implies a dualism, but not quite the dualism that Latour imputes to the 'moderns'. Rather, my position implies a dualism of science as a practice, with its own theories and approaches on the one hand, and society, with its many other practices, theories, and approaches on the other hand. This dualism relies upon (perhaps one would say it is an expression of) an idea that is now quite commonly held, to wit that science is to an important degree an independent endeavour. Peter Wilson says it is 'independent and universal' (2004, p. 59). By independent, I understand Wilson to mean that it has its own descriptive and explanatory resources (an idea expressed also by Ian Chalmers). So, it is not merely a disguised form of some other endeavour, for example politics (this is contrary to sceptical claims about psychiatry such as those of Szasz). Whether it is universal is perhaps a moot point. I would not, for example, want to claim that everyone has to accept the medical approach, that it is universal in that sense. But all I have to claim is that medical science, as a science, has its own descriptive and explanatory resources in terms of which it constructs its objects. This is an idea I mooted in the previous chapter, and I shall want to appeal to it and enlarge upon it here.

Attention deficit hyperactivity disorder as a medical (illness) category

In this chapter, the term ADHD is taken to refer to a medical approach to what is claimed to be a recognizable pattern of behaviours. This pattern of behaviours consists of problems with paying attention, control of impulses, and hyperactivity. It is suggested that this is a fairly stable triad (cf. Accardo and Blondis, 2000). It is to be seen in various forms in most of the recent DSM descriptions. In DSM-IV (American Psychiatric Association, 1994) this pattern of behaviours is itself named ADHD. But whenever I use the term ADHD I shall have in mind the medical account of these behaviours, that is to say the medical explanation of why and how they occur. To refer to the behaviours themselves I will use the term ADHD behaviours.

It would, however, be misleading to claim that ADHD is synonymous with a single medical account or explanation that is accepted by all. Current medical thinking about the nature of ADHD remains divided in certain important respects.

> In recent years, the accuracy of the term ADHD has been questioned by several researchers as individuals with ADHD do not seem to show prominent deficits in attention as it is defined and measured in the field of neuropsychology. Instead, deficits are most prominent in the appropriate linking of incoming information to a response, response inhibition, timing, and pacing. Mercugliano (2000, p. 62; see also Barkley, 1997, p. 8)

Mercugliano's comment refers to one of the major divides in the literature about ADHD. For example, Blondis *et al.* (2000) focus on the measurement of attention, while Barkley (1997) thinks it is a problem of self-control (inhibition of response). A review of the history of the idea reveals that historically earlier conceptualizations have also differed substantially (Conrad, 1976; Accardo and Blondis, 2000; Singh, 2002). There have also been moves to separate the diagnostic category into various subgroups (reflected for example in the appearance of both ADHD and ADD in DSM-IIIR: cf. Barkley, 1997, p. 7). Barkley suggests, for example, that one of the subgroups implicit in DSM-IV may have a qualitatively different mode of attention deficit (Barkley, 1997, p. 9).

However, these differences about the exact nature of ADHD should not hide what is a shared basic form to the understanding which characterizes ADHD. For the purposes of this chapter, this shared basic form can be summed up under two broad aspects. (1) ADHD is explicable in terms of a particular psychological characteristic—an essential nature, perhaps we could call it, in the form of a psychological construct, in terms of which the behaviours can be understood, and (2) ADHD involves a brain area or process causally associated with this psychological construct or nature. This brain area is in some way abnormal. This basic form echoes the form that has been taken to mark out a medical approach throughout the foregoing chapters. In what follows, I shall take it that to claim that someone has ADHD is simply to claim that an account with this form will be appropriate to its explanation and understanding. This is not to say that any medical account of ADHD must take this form: medicine moves on and may produce all sorts of forms of explanation in the future. However, current medicine certainly tends to explanations of behavioural problems that take the form I have described here. To illustrate specific examples of this form in ADHD, I shall most frequently refer to Barkley's theory, but this should not be taken to suggest that I believe Barkley's is the best or the right theory.

From the point of view of the kind of sceptical social constructionist critique I shall be offering, the fundamental point about the medical form of explanation just described is that it involves locating the problem ADHD represents with or in the individual. This is also fundamental to a problem that I shall have with supporting my position against the social constructionist while at the same time advancing my metaphor view of ADHD. For individualization appears fundamental to the medical approach: which means that on my account it appears to come with or be part and parcel of the metaphor of ADHD. To seek to understand behaviours in terms of ADHD is at the very least to seek to understand them in terms of the individual. However, the social constructionist sceptic argues that this is individualization and so reveals or unmasks it as in effect a political or social move. Note that the claim here is not that it is merely the reproduction of such a move, as the strong programme in the sociology of knowledge would say, and which it has in my view significant problems in showing (see Chapter 6). Rather, individualization is a political or social move in and of itself. This apparently makes the metaphor a political or social move. Yet I want to claim that psychiatry as a medical science is not politics, that it is in some sense independent of social practices of that ilk.

7.2 What is social construction?

I have suggested that social constructionism is an approach, rather than a programme, and that it may lead to the sceptical claim about ADHD that it is a social construct and hence does not have the reality it claims to have. I have also suggested that its method is historical.[1] I have also contrasted it implicitly with the strong programme in the sociology of knowledge, discussed in the previous chapter. Here I want to go further into this contrast. I shall suggest that both the strong programme and the social constructionist approach rest upon an historical approach. However, I shall suggest that it is the social constructionist who is able more effectively to turn this into a sceptical move.

A fundamental similarity: the historical approach

The historical approach was well illustrated in the previous chapter. I gave a history of the emergence of mental illness in the nineteenth century, which involved the role of the belief in the values of capitalism. In the light of this belief, so the history went, individuals were regarded as productive units. This view of individuals was naturalized, that is to say it was claimed to be the nature of human individuals to be productive. In the words of Douglas, a social category was reproduced as a supposedly a priori and necessary category (that is to say, a category of the sort that would be found in nature). In the light of this, the failure to be productive was presented as an unnatural state. However, some non-productivity was said to be the result of other apparently natural forces that were understood as making some individuals incapable of being productive. This idea was construed as the basis of the claim that the existence of mental illness was relative to—contingent upon—the view that people are productive units, and the social beliefs that engendered this view, namely capitalism. Mental illness was posited as a natural force to explain why some people did not act as they naturally should. In the argument I put forward in the previous chapter, this in turn led to an implicit contrast between mental illness and the supposed natural (non-socially contingent) existence of physical illnesses. Given that the existence of mental illness appeared to be contingent upon historical forces its reality was called into doubt.

The historical approach, then, broadly involves identifying a narrative of a particular kind to explain apparently natural categories. The particular kind of narrative to which the historical turn draws attention involves the social aspects of human existence. History in the historical approach is, in effect, a social history, involving the sorts of forces we understand as characterizing society. There are of course philosophical and theoretical differences about what does characterize society and social history. However, I shall take it that human beliefs, ideas, values, social institutions, movements, political ideals, and so on dominate this kind of narrative. It deals in things that are the product of humans.

Initially at least a social constructionist account of ADHD pursues a similar course to that of the strong programme. Hacking argues that the point of social constructionism is to combat a perceived naturalness or inevitability in the current state of affairs. Its aim is to show that an apparently natural or inevitable feature of or idea about either our world or our minds is after all a historical, a human, product. That is, its aim is to show how the social forces enshrined in beliefs, institutions, social movements, political parties, and so on have produced or constructed this thing. This implies, Hacking points out, that unless there is an initial perception that the feature or idea in question is unavoidable or natural, social constructionism is otiose. For example, he notes that there is no point in developing and trying to prove a thesis that something such as the British monarchy has social origins, as it would be odd to doubt it in the first place. The British monarchy, he says, is clearly an institution of society and not inevitable in any way (Hacking, 1999, p. 12). Hacking may be forgetting that the British Monarchy once saw itself in a rather different light namely as divinely ordained by God to rule, but waiving that, Hacking's point is well taken. The belief that the feature or idea is a natural or unavoidable aspect of the world is 'a precondition for a social constructionist thesis' about that feature or idea (p. 12).

ADHD meets this precondition: it represents itself, in its very conception, as a biological product, rather than a human, social product. It can be argued, against this, that it is described in DSM, for example, in behavioural terms, and that no comment is made about its origins or nature. However, it is widely

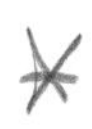

agreed that DSM represents its behavioural descriptions as signs of underlying physical pathology. And the whole research thrust of ADHD is towards functions and the brain. So, like the strong programme in the sociology of knowledge, social constructionism seeks to show how something that is presented as a feature of the biological (the brain most obviously) is in fact the product of a human, historical, social story.

Differences

There are, however, a number of significant differences between the strong programme and a social constructionist approach. These relate to the conclusions at which they drive, based on their historical analyses. For the strong programme, in reality, is not sceptical in the way social constructionist accounts can be. I adapted, or sought to adapt, the strong programme to a sceptical account of mental illness. This involved, as I mentioned just above, presenting the argument that mental illness arose relative to the capitalist idea that people are naturally productive units. This in turn was directed towards the sceptical conclusion that psychiatry was a pseudo-science. Mental illness, the supposed strong programme argument was supposed to be, does not have the reality of physical illnesses because it is the product of history, so the branch of medicine that claims to treat it is also a product of history and can claim no sounder foundation than history offers. History does not offer a very stable footing, as history is among other things a story of change, and any particular historical setting is likely to be temporary in some or all of its lineaments.

But in reality, as I also mentioned in the last chapter, the strong programme is not adaptable to such specific or targeted scepticism about things. This is because the strong programme is not targeted. It is, rather, a general account of the apparently natural and sometimes logical categories of things that appear in all knowledge and belief. For example, as I mentioned, its proponents have turned their attention to mathematics (in particular to numbers), to Newtonian corpuscles and also to philosophical theories, notably those in the philosophy of science. Newton's corpuscular theories were said to be a reproduction of his religious ideas; Kuhn's and Popper's contrasting philosophies of science seemed to reproduce their different political ideals (Bloor, 1976, p. 65, 1982a; and Chapter 6). In fact there is in principle no limit to the sciences and other disciplines to which the strong programme is applicable. If the conclusion of the strong programme was the one I sought to adapt it to in the case of psychiatry—i.e. that psychiatry was a pseudo-science—it would follow by the same token that all sciences were pseudo-sciences. But this is a paradoxical conclusion: if all so-called sciences are pseudo-sciences, then there is no contrast between science and pseudo-science, and hence nothing can be either a science or a pseudo-science. In fact, the strong programme aims to break down the distinction between pseudo and authentic sciences. A common way of putting this distinction has been to hold that pseudo-sciences reflect the interests of their practitioners and those whose social interests are bound up with their practice (e.g. Lysenko's anti-Darwinian beliefs fitted Soviet Marxist political perspectives), and retain their status only through social means (e.g. Lysenko's influence survives through support of the Communist Party). The strong programme seeks to show that this much is true of all sciences.

A social constructionist approach, however, as Hacking suggests, is able to take a sceptical line on something as specific as ADHD (or mental illness, for example) because it can be targeted. It can do this because (and to the extent that) it does preserve the distinction between natural categories and categories that are presented as natural but are in fact created through human agency and perhaps for human purposes. Given this, it can target particular sciences or enterprises within science, and make a number of different levels of criticism of them, including the sort of outright scepticism about psychiatry or particular diagnoses within it that I am interested in. In doing so, social constructionists can take up what Hacking calls a reformist line: they can seek to persuade people that ADHD is not merely a human product, but one that society would be better off without. In what follows I shall assume that getting rid of the very idea of ADHD is the aim of the sceptical social constructionist critique: it is certainly the aim of Breggin for example, and I think of writers such as Timimi too (cf. Timimi and Taylor, 2004).

The mode of criticism I shall be most interested in is indeed a sceptical one in this sense. Hacking calls it unmasking. This is one of a number of what he calls metaphors which he uses in describing social constructionism, taking this one from the work of Mannheim. The 'unmasking turn of mind', Hacking cites Mannheim as saying, is

> a turn of mind which does not seek to refute, negate, or call in doubt certain ideas, but rather to *disintegrate* them, and that in such a way that the whole world outlook of a social stratum becomes disintegrated at the same time. We must pay attention, at this point, to the phenomenological distinction between 'denying the truth' of an idea, and 'determining the function' it exercises. In denying the truth of an idea, I still presuppose it as 'thesis' and thus put myself upon the same theoretical (and nothing but theoretical) basis as the one on which the idea is constituted. In casting doubt upon the 'idea,' I still think within the same categorical pattern as the one in which it has its being. But when I do not even raise the question (or at least when I do not make this question the burden of my argument) whether what the idea asserts is true, but consider it merely in terms of the *extra-theoretical function* it serves, then, and only then, do I achieve an 'unmasking' which in fact represents no theoretical refutation but the destruction of the practical effectiveness of these ideas. Mannheim (1952, p. 140; cited in Hacking, 1999, pp. 52–3)

Several things are of particular relevance in Mannheim's words to what follows, and I will just take a moment to pick them out and say something about them now: (1) the focus on an *idea*; (2) the notion of the *extratheoretical function* of an idea; and (3) the distinction between *unmasking* and *refuting* and the idea of *disintegration* of an idea.

The focus on the idea

The focus being on ideas links directly into a sociological analysis that plays such an important role in the social constructionist approach, but which social constructionism goes beyond. Describing the sociological approach to illness and health care, Conrad (who is an early social constructivist critic of ADHD though not altogether a sceptic) quotes Friedson: 'From the sociological point of view . . . the problem to manage is the *idea* of illness itself—*how signs and symptoms get to be labeled or diagnosed as illness* in the first place, how an individual gets to be labeled sick and how social behavior is molded by the process of diagnosis and treatment.' (Friedson, 1970, p. 212 Conrad's emphasis; cited in Conrad, 1976, p. 52).

In Friedson's sociological analysis, illness is an idea. This implies, *inter alia*, that it is not an intrinsic property of any condition of the human person. Rather, one is *said to be* or perhaps *declared* ill (one has illness attributed to one). Certain people—medically trained doctors in Western societies—are given the authority by society to do this declaring. And if one is declared ill or sick, one enters what an earlier sociologist (Parsons) called 'the sick role'. One may then be legitimated in acting in a certain way, taking time off work for example; and may be expected to seek and comply with treatment. This role constitutes the sociological meaning of the category or idea of illness—its social meaning, impact, or function.

A sociological analysis of ADHD starts, then, with this sort of insight: ADHD is an idea with a social meaning, impact, and function. The sociological task, a la Friedson, would be to understand that function of the idea of ADHD.

Extratheoretical function of ideas

Mannheim argues that ideas have functions that are extratheoretical. (He also talks of 'supra-theoretical factors' that condition thought. Cf. 1952, p. 137.) I understand Mannheim to be implying a contrast between this extratheoretical function of an idea on the one hand, and on the other hand the sort of role that idea plays when we understand it in its own terms and in the context of the 'categorial pattern . . . in which it has its being'. For example, in its own terms, ADHD is a medical diagnosis, and is one of a number of such diagnoses. It is understood in the way other medical diagnoses are understood, and in the medical world it is assumed to refer to a state of the human psychology/brain that is an object of treatment, research, and medical congresses. This is the 'theoretical' function of the idea of ADHD. So, clearly Mannheim's notion of extratheoretical function refers to some other function than this.

This is also what Friedson's idea of illness does: it refers to a function other than that the idea of illness plays within medicine. However, to understand what Mannheim means by extratheoretical function of an idea, we have to contrast it with the sociological function of which Friedson writes. The difference between Friedson's idea of an extratheoretical function and Mannheim's lies in the disintegrating purpose to which Mannheim puts it. Friedson does not see identification of the sociological function of an idea such as illness as in any way undermining its medical function. So even though, in some sense, the sociological function Friedson identifies is extratheoretical—its meaning is not determined by the medical understanding of the term illness and can be understood independently of it—the existence of this function does not unmask the medical notion, but coexists with it.

Hacking gives an example of the extratheoretical function of the kind he takes Mannheim to have in mind in looking at the idea of the 'serial killer'. The extratheoretical function of this category might be 'to serve certain interests, and to gratify certain fantasies' Hacking suggests. It is perhaps 'intended to deflect attention from gun-control, inner city mayhem . . .' (1999, p. 55). Taking this at face value for a moment (Hacking is offering a token analysis, not one he has worked out in detail or sought to prove) the argument would be that the category serial killer has been invented for (right-wing?) political purposes. It suits the right-wing political agenda to focus public concerns about violence on a few isolated and highly deviant individuals rather than on the free availability of guns in society more generally. In the same spirit, with respect to ADHD, the social constructionist who seeks to unmask and disintegrate it is looking for interests, fantasies, and/or whatever political purposes the idea of ADHD may serve.

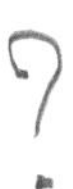

Unmasking not refuting

Once we see what we can broadly call the political purposes for which the category has been invented, Mannheim says, we have disintegrated or dissolved the idea. In doing this, questions such as 'Is there an increase in the numbers of serial-killers?' (to take up Hacking's example again), which imply taking the category seriously, become otiose or by-the-way. Likewise, in the case of ADHD, one of the questions that Cannon *et al.* mention 'Is the incidence of ADHD rising?' would become tangential, a diversion.

But at first sight it is not clear why an idea should be disintegrated just because one identifies a function that it has outside the one it seems to fit in with theoretically. If ADHD is theoretically speaking a medical idea, but extratheoretically (say sociologically speaking) a gateway to certain kinds of special treatment or funding (a la Friedson's analysis), why not simply admit it is both? This is indeed precisely what Friedson does.

To understand what Mannheim may have in mind, it is useful to note that he compares unmasking with calling someone a liar. Though he thinks there is a clear difference between them, the similarity is more significant for our purposes at this point. (Later the difference will prove to be vital.) Mannheim says that calling someone a liar is not necessarily to say they have said an untruth. When we call someone a liar 'what we say concerns rather a certain relation of the subject making the utterance to the proposition it expresses . . . we consider statements of a subject from the point of view of his ethical personality' (1952, pp. 140–1). An example might be saying that a psychiatrist diagnoses ADHD in order to retain his or her power and prestige within society. The relation of this subject to his/her propositions is that claims such as 'you have ADHD' are motivated by the importance of the profession, and do not represent an expression of a genuine medical judgement. Or we might remember the story of Matilda who called the fire brigade when there was no fire. When there really was a fire, people took an unmasking approach to her cries of 'fire' and focusing on her ethical personality 'only shouted "little liar"' (Belloc, 1970, pp. 262–4).

By disintegration Mannheim refers to an attitude towards ideas that has as its upshot 'the destruction of the practical effectiveness of these ideas' (p. 140). In taking an unmasking attitude to Matilda's cries ('fire!') their practical effectiveness (which should have been to secure help to rescue her from the burning house) was indeed destroyed. The equivalent in the case of ADHD would make it impossible to pursue it within its apparent theoretical realm: every claim to diagnose it would be greeted with the same reaction, namely that it serves the social and political interests of psychiatrists.

Mannheim notes that the difference between unmasking in the case of calling someone a liar and unmasking in the sense he has in mind is primarily that the subject (the psychiatric profession, Matilda 'who told lies and was burned to death') becomes 'an impersonal socio-intellectual force' (p. 141). This will prove to be a fundamentally important distinction later on: when Mannheim uses this phrase he has in mind ideologies or 'the world outlook of a social stratum' (p. 140). Hacking argues that social constructionism can be seen to unmask at a point somewhere between these two. That is to say, as mentioned earlier, social constructionism can pick and choose fairly specific targets. It does not have to unmask whole 'world outlooks'. It also means that we can identify different examples of such socio-political forces. It does not need to be something as broad a class or social stratum.

In the next section, I will set out what I take to be a possible—and I think a powerful—social constructionist account of ADHD, trying to show how it would seek to unmask it.

7.3 A social constructionist critique of attention deficit hyperactivity disorder

So, how does one unmask an idea such as ADHD? I shall suggest an unmasking social constructionist approach modelled on that of Conrad. Conrad presents his arguments in the case of what was then called hyperkinesis; however, they can be applied to ADHD. I use Conrad for several reasons: Though his critique is rather old chronologically, it remains one of the most thorough (and Conrad has continued to write in the area since). Furthermore, Conrad's critique is one of the most challenging for my position. It is Conrad who identifies the role of individualization in the medical form that characterizes ADHD.

Conrad's argument about hyperkinesis adapted to ADHD would be that it represents the de-politicization of an issue.

> [B]y defining the overactive, restless, and disruptive child as hyperkinetic we ignore the meaning of behavior in the context of the social system. If we focused our analysis on the school system we might see the child's behavior as symptomatic of some 'disorder' in the school or classroom situation . . . In this sense it [medicalisation] is similar to the individualisation of social problems, only the focus is different. Rather than focusing on the social problem the notion of depoliticisation focuses on the meaning of behavior. . . . We render the deviant behavior, which might actually be a form of social conflict, meaningless. How much do these children have to tell us about the school system, the family situation and our society itself? Conrad (1976, p. 75)

This expresses the extratheoretical function of the idea of hyperkinesis. It turns out to be somewhat like Hacking's off-the-cuff example of the idea of the serial killer. It is a smoke screen, if you like, hiding other agendas from view. Just as the idea of the serial killer diverts attention from the social dangers of widespread gun ownership by making it look as though murders are basically down to certain maverick and perverted individuals, so the idea of ADHD diverts attention from social problems in the child's social context (what Conrad calls disorder in the school or classroom). It focuses instead on the children who it might be said merely register those contextual disorders. The wider agenda that is hidden in this is the tendency of modern US society (the setting of Conrad's analysis) to foster the individual as the basic building block of society, and to deny the existence or importance of supra-individual institutions.

So the social constructionist position I am interested in expounding needs to show that two things are happening in the case of ADHD. One is that there is a social context in which ADHD behaviours become an issue, and the other is that the idea of ADHD hides this by locating the problem in the individual rather than in the context. I shall focus more on the second: this is for two reasons. First, establishing that there is a social context in which ADHD behaviours become an issue is something that is already regularly done in the literature: indeed, it seems to be something there is little one can do to deny. Second, even when we have established that there is an ineradicable social context to ADHD, we do not arrive at unmasking. So the work remains to be done in showing how the idea of ADHD focuses on the individual and so becomes functional extratheoretically.

The social context of attention deficit hyperactivity disorder behaviours

In one sense, there is little or no argument that ADHD behaviours must exist in some social context. However, the problem is to show what follows from this: I shall argue that it does not necessarily lead to unmasking.

Widely accepted descriptions of ADHD behaviours—such as that in DSM-IV—are clearly normative, which is to say they reflect various social values. They contain phrases such as 'often leaves seat in classroom or other situations in which remaining seated is expected' in which the norms are explicit. These phrases cannot successfully be expunged from the description: it relies upon them. For example, if we remove the norms in this criterion of ADHD (which is (b) under the hyperactivity axis) we are left with 'often leaves seat' (provided, that is, that often is not also seen as inviting a normative judgement—i.e. *too* often). Clearly, if we place this description in the context of a crowded bus, in which the child regularly gives up his or her place to other more needy passengers, we do not have a description that invites explanation in disease terms.

We can also identify slightly wider norms within which these more specific ideas emerge. Through the criteria around inattention for example, the ADHD child appears as the shadow of an ideal child, who is attentive to details, careful with whatever tasks he/she is given (criterion a) gives sustained attention (b) listens when spoken to (c) follows through on instructions and finishes whatever tasks he/she is given (d) is good at organizing her or himself to get things done (e). This child is little trouble in the classroom or at home as he/she is willing to 'engage in tasks that require sustained mental effort' (f). DSM is based upon many years of observation and expert opinion (see Barkley, 1997, p. 14), but this does not prevent these observations reflecting such powerful values.

There is certainly, at first sight, a route from this to the claim that ADHD does not exist in the way it is supposed by scientists, doctors, and indeed many sufferers, to exist. Conrad suggests that the normative basis of the description means that at the bottom of hyperkinesis there is a social judgement of deviance. Of this he says:

> This perspective considers deviance not as inherent to the individual, the act, or the situation, but rather as a process in which certain alleged 'rule-breaking' actions come to be defined as deviance and certain individual rule breakers become labeled as deviant. The emphasis is on the societal reaction to the act or behavior, not on the act or behavior itself. In an early elaboration of this perspective Howard S. Becker stated, 'In short whether an act is deviant or not depends in part on the nature of the act (that is, whether or not it violates some rule) and in part on what other people do about it' (1963:14). As Kai Erikson put it, deviance is attributed to action: 'Deviance is not a property *inherent* in any particular kind of behavior; it is a property *conferred upon* that behavior by people who come into direct or indirect contact with it' (1966:6). Conrad (1976, p. 1)

What might appear to lead on to a sceptical conclusion in this account is the idea that deviance is not inherent in the behaviour. It is conferred upon or attributed to it by third parties (although, in the case of adult ADHD, we would need to acknowledge that among those who confer the property are those who claim that they have ADHD and so confer it on themselves). It appears that in denying that the deviance lies in any property of the behaviour itself, Conrad sets the groundwork for a potential sceptical denial of the illness explanation of ADHD behaviours.

This groundwork of scepticism would lie in the idea that ADHD behaviours exist only in the light of social values of some sort. Its existence, it might be argued, is relative to those values. Where they do not exist, neither do the behaviours. And as values reflect an historical or cultural state, it is likely that they will pass away at some point, taking ADHD with them. This, it can be supposed, is not the way one would expect things to be if the behaviours were produced by a biological feature of the individual—which would be what the medical perspective would claim lay beneath the behaviours. This appears to suggest an extratheoretical role, in that ADHD must be something other than the illness it claims to be.

However, this argument can plausibly be countered by the claim of the proponent of ADHD that the descriptions in DSM-IV are only the beginning of the issue. They can argue that these accounts are untheorized (cf. Barkley, 1997) and that it remains to be seen whether effective theoretical accounts can be given of them. If this is right then we cannot altogether avoid the theoretical level at which ADHD operates by going along this route: the argument that ADHD behaviours are identified only in virtue of norms does not lead directly to an extratheoretical account.

A further problem with the argument from the normative nature of descriptions of ADHD behaviours is that it shadows the sort of approach used in the previous chapter. It suggests that ADHD is actually a social or moral category, which is reproduced in an apparently natural category. As we argued in the previous chapter, there is a difficulty making out the claim that a moral category can be reproduced in biological terms. Insofar as the first account relies upon this idea of reproduction, it will run up against similar problems: it will be difficult to see how moral criteria ('Often leaves seat [when] remaining seated is expected') can be reproduced in medical criteria.

While the claim that ADHD behaviours reflect values in their social context is clearly true, this does not necessarily lead to unmasking ADHD.

Attention deficit hyperactivity disorder and individualization

We have established that ADHD behaviours are identified in normative terms. They exist rather as crime (or criminals) exist: that is to say as the result of a certain kind of judgement, which is expressed in rules or laws of conduct. In the case of ADHD, the judgement seems to relate to a comparison with an ideal child, and the points of this comparison are expressed in the criteria found in DSM for example. As with the case of crime, without these criteria of description, the behaviours that are identified in terms of those criteria, must be absent.

However, I have also suggested that there is a potential response from the proponent of ADHD. It is that the attribution of deviance is a starting point, but is not the full story. Rather, the existence of deviance raises a question about why the person is acting in what is perceived as a deviant manner. And it can be argued that deviant behaviour is explicable in medical terms. This is not to say that all deviant behaviour can be explained in this way: this was Szasz's fear ('the medicalisation of morality') and something that Anthony Flew (1973) argued against in his book *Crime or Disease*? But it is to accept that it is possible to explain some behaviour in this way.

Notwithstanding, I shall suggest that a social constructionist might seek to argue that because of the nature of ADHD—that is to say the fact that the idea takes a medical form—it is by its very nature social. To diagnose ADHD, and indeed to produce the very idea of ADHD, is a social or, it might be said, a political act. It is a political act just because it locates the problem in the individual rather than in society. Indeed, a similar argument can in theory be mounted about mental illness in general, and about any other particular diagnosis or diagnostic category. The whole idea of mental illness, it could be said, takes a range of behaviours that are socially difficult and says the problem lies in the individuals. This potential social constructionist argument is a problem for my position. I claim that ADHD implies a metaphor (the categorization of a set of behaviours as an illness). It appears, on the argument I shall be considering, that this is vehicle of the individualization. To categorize something as an illness is, at the very minimum, to say that the problem lies in one place (the person) rather than another (his or her social context).

And this would seem to be equivalent to setting the scene for unmasking it: it is to invite the possibility of diverting attention from the question whether so-and-so has ADHD, or from the question what kind of thing ADHD is, to the question of what motivates the idea of ADHD or its application. The question the unmasker asks is: Why this focus on the individual, rather than the social context? This is the sort of question Conrad's account of the individualization inherent in the idea of hyperactivity can be said to respond to:

> We tend to look for causes and solutions to complex social problems in the individual rather than in the social system. In some senses this resembles William Ryan's (1971) notion of 'blaming the victim'; seeing the causes of the problems in the individuals (who are usually of low status) rather than in the society in which they live. We then seek to change the 'victim' rather than the society. This is probably very consistent with the American dominant value system, which tends to emphasize the individual while minimizing the importance and influence of the community. The medical perspective of diagnosing an illness in an individual lends itself to the individualization of social problems. That is, rather than seeing certain deviant behaviors as symptomatic of problems in the social system, it focuses on the individual diagnosing and treating the illness, generally ignoring the social situation. Conrad (1976, pp. 74–5)

How might this approach apply to ADHD in detail? That the idea of ADHD takes a medical form is not difficult to argue. I suggested earlier that this form can be seen to have two aspects: a psychological essence of some kind and a causal account in terms of brain abnormalities that are taken to explain the psychological problems. Given that this is the basic structure of ADHD it is easy to see why it may be said to be an individualizing move. It does not seek an explanation of a child's or an adult's inability to pay attention or impulsivity in the face of extended mental tasks (for example) in the nature of the tasks set or the wider context (of school, home, or workplace) in which they are set. Rather it focuses on the individual psychology of the child or adult, and through that upon the individual's brain.

Barkley's theory of ADHD illustrates these two aspects of the medical form particularly clearly. I shall not go into Barkley's theory in detail—partly because it is complex and worked out at great length in its full form (cf. Barkley, 1997). However, it is important to see how, in terms of specifics, such theories represent the individual as the locus of the problem. Furthermore, it will be important to my approach to the way in which metaphor makes mental illnesses such as ADHD to see how it is that Barkley constructs or creates his evidence in the light of the way in which he categorizes ADHD behaviours as an illness.

Barkley conceptualizes the problem the individual has in functional terms. For him, psychologically (or perhaps we should say neuropsychologically) speaking, ADHD is a problem of self-control or, more specifically, inhibition. Barkley understands self-control to be produced by the cooperative working of five functions of the mind. To simplify—not too horribly I hope—one of these, inhibition, works in various ways to give space to the others (which include memory and which Barkley calls executive functions) to operate. Self-control then results in a person being able to weigh up the pros and cons of taking what is immediately on offer against what else might be on offer in the future. The weighting people give to the immediate against the long-term changes in part as people develop. However, in ADHD the functioning of the inhibition and of some of the executive functions is compromised. This, it is said, explains the impulsivity of those who exhibit ADHD behaviours, and their inability to work through mental tasks and why they are always getting off their seats when they are expected to sit still and concentrate. The sort of weighing or calculation that Barkley has in mind in self-control is between time and reward value. If the self-control functions are operating as they should, then the person takes into account greater reward value that might accrue by waiting compared with lesser, though more immediately available reward value. Barkley seems to think that the inability to do this is explained by the dysfunctioning of the inhibition, which then leaves the executive functions no time to come up with a calculation or present the person with alternative courses of action.

Barkley's account represents individualization, because once one sees an issue of this kind in terms of functions of the human mind, a rather different sort of account of what is going on is ruled out. This is the kind of account that treats the choice for the immediate reward as indicating a *preference* over the reward for which one has to wait, or a different evaluation of the supposed discounting of time against gain. In this kind of account, unlike in the function account, what we see is a difference of judgement. That is to say, the function account means that we do not have to face up to the possibility that someone has valued things differently.

It may be argued that an account that explains apparently impulsive behaviour in terms of different evaluations made by the person (child or adult) is no less an individualizing account than is the ADHD account that posits a psychological function to explain the behaviour. In either case, it may be thought, the problem is identified with the person rather than with the person's environment. However, the distinctive feature of the different values account is that it automatically raises questions about what the correct evaluation is. In other words, as Conrad argues, taken as a choice that reflects distinct values, ADHD behaviours suggest a criticism of or at least an alternative to the usually accepted evaluations. This meaning, it may be argued, is not conscious in the child, but it may still be taken to represent a different vision of what a child may be like. Different, that is, to the ideal that DSM-IV appears to express. In this way, it reintroduces the normative element and hence the social element that the function/dysfunction account sought to get away from.

The point that is being made here is very like one made earlier when we were considering the strong objection to the likeness argument. A functional account of behaviours, while it may be possible and indeed plausible, is only one possibility. We do not have to see the mental aspects of people in functional terms, though we can do. Barkley's ADHD account presupposes that a functional account is the correct one to give of the behaviours identified in DSM-IV and indeed elsewhere. It is not a conclusion from evidence. What it represents is the application of ADHD, the categorizing of the behaviours in illness terms. That is to say, the functional account is not independent of the idea that the behaviours in question are symptoms of an illness of some sort.

A riposte does seem to be available to Barkley and to other proponents of ADHD. This is that there is good evidence of brain abnormalities that accompany the behaviours. Barkley's theories for example speculate on what parts of the brain may be implicated in ADHD. He says that the executive functions that are components of self-control 'seem to be localized to the orbital-prefrontal regions and associated interconnections to the striatum'. He notes 'accumulating evidence' that interference control or 'persistent inhibition or resistance to distraction' (one of the forms that inhibition may take) 'may be somewhat more lateralized to the right anterior prefrontal region' and that inhibition of the decision to respond is 'situated in the orbital-prefrontal region' (Barkley, 1997, p. 156).

A problem for this kind of speculation, which arises in the light of the previous argument about the choice to see ADHD as a mental dysfunction of some form, is that it makes sense only in the light of that choice. The point at stake here is a large one: it is similar to a point that Canguilhem (1991) makes when it comes to the notion of the pathological. Canguilhem argues that we only come to the body in disease through a series of investigations of it when the person has already been identified as ill. We then call what we find a pathology. The pathological, which is a subject of medical science, is always secondary to a social judgement that someone is unwell. In the same vein, one can argue that the proposed dysfunctions of the mental in ADHD are secondary upon prior judgements that we have a medical problem (an illness) here. If we do not think of illness in the face of ADHD behaviours, then we will not explain those behaviours in illness (e.g. functional) terms. We would not appeal to dysfunction to explain variations in normative judgements. It can then be argued that theoretical discussion of what parts of the brain might be involved in ADHD are clearly not independent of the idea that ADHD behaviours represent an illness.

However, independently of theoretical discussion of what parts and systems of the brain may be involved in ADHD, there have been studies of brain activity through various modes of neuroimaging. The significance accorded to neuroimaging studies of ADHD is very great. Accardo and Blondis, giving a history of ADHD say that 'The now classic study by Zametkin *et al.* (1990) finally settled the issue of the existence of an organic basis to ADHD as a syndrome' (2000, p. 7). Zametkin used a PET (positron emission tomography) scanner to look at global glucose metabolism in different areas of the brains those said to have ADHD and a control group. The study showed significant differences in areas such as the prefrontal and premotor cortex (Sieg, 2000, p. 99). Clearly, if this is a correct interpretation of the raw data, it can be argued that the scanner proves this significance to whoever cares to look at it. It does not show one thing to the person who espouses ADHD and another to the social constructionist unmasker.

A standard reply from a sceptical angle would be to say that the direction of causality is unclear. Perhaps, it may be argued, the so-called abnormal brain readings are the result of mental states that accompany behaviours that are disvalued, such as leaving one's seat too often or failing to do one's homework. However, I want to make a related point in a slightly different way.

This starts with the observation that metabolic measures (such as PET scans) 'average over relatively large volumes of tissue' and so obscure judgements at a more detailed level. For example, Lock and Bender, who take it that ADHD is an attentional problem, argue that the there is a 'push-pull nature of attentional modulation that is evident at single neuron level'. This is a reference to experimental findings that where attention is being paid, at the neuronal level some neurones respond more while others respond less (Lock and Bender, 2000, p. 37). Clearly, if, as a matter of fact, attention involves some areas doing more and other areas doing less, an average of all this neuronal activity hides this. A landscape of peaks and valleys is, when averaged out, an unvarying plain. This means that the measurements cannot distinguish between a plain that is the product of the averaging, and a plain that is actually a plain—a person in whom there are no pushes or pulls.

As this stands, it is no more than an observation about what PET scans can show at the neuronal level. But Lock and Bender's point can be developed at a wider level. Their point in the specific case is that what a measure of some kind in ADHD means is not to be discovered free of some theory about, for example, attention at the neuronal level. At the wider level, the point is that measurements of brain activity through scans reveal their meaning only in virtue of particular theoretical approaches ready to interpret the data. And this can be seen to be a close cousin to the claim that the meaning of what is measured is not to be discovered free of pre-existing ideas. That is to say, what PET scans reveal is not to be understood independently of the claim that some brains have ADHD. This, then introduces the idea of ADHD as an essential part in the interpretation of PET scan data. Only with this idea already in mind does such data yield conclusions about, for example, the causes of a psychological dysfunction.

In other words, even though it may be claimed that the neuroimaging data is observable independently of the idea that ADHD behaviours are symptomatic of an illness (namely ADHD), what those data might mean—how they are to be interpreted—entails the use of some conceptualization or other. If these arguments are right, ADHD cannot be said to be supported by brain evidence. Brain evidence cannot be taken to dictate to the observer what it means. Rather, the sort of data Zametkin *et al.* have come up with can be said to represent evidence of an organic basis of ADHD when it is already categorized in illness terms. Categorized this way evidence emerges that an illness explains what is going on. In short it represents the metaphor of mental illness.

But, and here's the rub for my argument, it also represents individualization. That is to say it appears to be a political move. To place ADHD under the category of illness is in effect to silence the behaviours as a criticism of society. This, at any rate, is what I think Conrad's account suggests. This is achieved by decoupling ADHD from the social: it is conceptualized as being without social meaning. This is precisely what functional and causal—i.e. illness—accounts do. They operate within a set of descriptive resources which work with biological or more narrowly medical concepts and connections. And this also suggests how ADHD may be unmasked. Using the descriptive resources of biology removes from the picture the possibility of social criticism. The silencing of social criticism suggests that there is something to defend. ADHD may be said to represent a diversion from the real problem.

7.4 The social constructionist account considered

The foregoing has brought together two things: the categorization of ADHD behaviours as a disease (i.e. as ADHD) and the notion of individualization as a political (that is to say a social) move. In diagnosing ADHD the psychiatrist is diverting attention from the social context in which the individual lives and focusing it upon the individual. This, or so it seems, can be construed as a political move. And in virtue of this, it seems to open the whole idea of ADHD up to a sceptical social constructionism that claims that this focus on the individual is the extratheoretical function of the idea. This is, according to Mannheim to unmask ADHD, that is to say render it ineffective in practical terms in its own theoretical area.

I shall argue that we are not committed to this unmasking.

Many who consider—and some who use—a social constructionist approach come to non-sceptical conclusions about ADHD. They do not go so far as to seek to unmask it. Singh focuses on a condition called emotional disturbance which is often claimed to be a precursor of ADHD at a slightly earlier period even than Conrad (i.e. the 1940–60s), but she applies her findings to ADHD itself. She describes her aim thus: 'I hope to make the point that as long as we understand ADHD to be a de-contextualized problem of an individual brain we miss seeing the social-scientific commitments that have been borne along in the ADHD diagnosis and in Ritalin treatment' (Singh, 2002, p. 580). Enlarging on the social scientific commitment, Singh identifies this as: 'the intimate association between a problem boy and his problematic mother. I suggest that this association has encouraged scientific interventions in childrearing generally, and more specifically, it has supported, and may continue to support, mothers' turn to ADHD diagnosis and Ritalin treatment for their children's behavior and performance' (p. 580).

This focus is in turn a feature of a wider worry about the health of America's youth. Singh sees in it a wider political concern, for the future and pre-eminence of democracy (see p. 583). Conrad might say the concern for democracy was in turn an expression of the belief in the individual, thus bringing Singh's theory in line with his own.

The important phrase for my purposes in Singh's words is 'borne along in'. This phrase implies the idea that the focus on the problem boy and his problem mother is expressed or ensconced in such ideas as that of emotional disturbance. But 'borne along in' does not suggest identity. Barges are borne along in the waters of the Rhine, yet there is clearly a distinction between them and the river waters. Conrad has a similar turn of phrase. He says that the focus on the individual in hyperactivity 'is probably *very consistent with* the American dominant value system, which tends to emphasize the individual while minimizing the importance and influence of the community' (1976, p. 73: my italics). That is to say, there is a fit between a medical approach (which focuses upon the individual) and an individualistic political approach. But what fits with individualistic politics is not necessarily just a branch of individualistic politics.

The point that Conrad and Singh can be seen to be making is well taken: clearly if medicine identifies problems in terms of the brain and psychology, it will individualize them. Therefore, it will fit in with an approach that says that the individual is the fundamental political or social building block. It is on a par with the relation between Newton's physical atoms acted upon by external forces and made to go which ever way those forces drove them, and his ideal society, in which individuals, atom-like, would be told what to believe by authorities external to them.

But just as clearly, what Conrad and Singh claim stops short of saying that fit is identity. Both think that the social context (the focus on the mother–child relationship and the inherent individualism of US society) is significant, but not that emotional disturbance or hyperkinesis (or ADHD) are nothing more than this focus.

Someone might argue that Conrad and Singh have stopped short when they should not have or at least did not have to. The argument might go like this:

> You hold that there is a fit between the medical approach and the political individualizing approach. However, in the case of ADHD, this is more than a fit. This is because in turning attention to the individual medically one is turning attention away from the context: one is diverting attention from the political, if you like, to the medical. But to divert attention from the political is a political move. To define ADHD as a medical problem (to categorize it that way) can be said to be a move in a political arena because it involves shifting arenas—it is, if you like, implicitly a decision between the arenas in question.

An initial response to this argument is that it is too powerful for its own good. If turning attention to the individual in an individualistic political context is sufficient to demonstrate an extratheoretical function, then very many more medical diagnoses than that of ADHD will be included. The social constructionist sceptic would then find his or her argument applying in places where it was not targeted. Potentially, especially if the sceptic wanted to apply it to all mental illnesses, for example, this might at first appear acceptable. However, it is not clear that its implications could be restricted to mental illnesses, or indeed even to illnesses. There are many cases where we identify a problem that could in theory be put down to the social context with an individual (crime comes to mind again, and perhaps immorality in general).

The problem here lies in the idea of sufficiency. What is needed is something to restrict the application of the social constructionist critique. One way of doing this would be to say that ADHD (or, if the argument was to be applied more generally, that mental illness) shows the individualization agenda particularly. For example, it could be argued that ADHD relies on behaviours in certain restricted social contexts and in the light of particular expectations (broadly speaking, educational institutions and academic achievements). In contrast, it could be said, other mental illnesses such as schizophrenia appear in behaviours identified in much less specific social contexts. A child with ADHD appears only in classrooms and in the context of high educational expectations such as those of middle class New Yorkers (or so it may be claimed); but those who claim to be Napoleon or that thoughts are being inserted into their heads by aliens would surely stand out in any context.

However, the narrowness of the context in which behaviours may appear is not a convincing means of restricting the application of the social constructionist critique. One reason for this is because in cases that the social constructionist might want to exclude from scepticism a similar narrowness may appear. Colour blindness, for example, may show only in very specific contexts. Indeed, it may be that many childhood problems will be revealed especially in schools (restricted hearing, short sight). However, the social constructionist sceptic about ADHD may well wish not to be sceptical about these. Conversely, theorizations of ADHD have suggested that it is a much broader problem than simply one of attending in classrooms, and that it is capable of showing in many places other than such restricted educational behavioural contexts. If, as Barkley argues, ADHD is a failure of self-control, then it presumably will show wherever self-control is an issue.

So, it appears that the social constructionist sceptic will have problems restricting scepticism to ADHD if the basis of his or her argument is the location of a problem in an individual, in a context in which the problem could be located in the social context, and in which individualism is a dominant political value.

The problem, I believe, arises because a distinction is being glossed over. Even if, as the social constructionist claims, ADHD represents the individualization of a problem it does not follow that the character of the individualization is determined by its extratheoretical function. This is the case even if we acknowledge that such an individualization may have an extratheoretical function. It is useful here to return to Mannheim's distinction between the idea of a lie and the idea of unmasking in the sociological sense. When someone is accused of being a liar our focus is on that person and his or her motivation (her 'ethical character' as Mannheim puts it). However, if our focus is on what he calls 'an impersonal socio-intellectual force' (1952, p. 141) then we have yet to determine what characterizes this.

This is precisely where the idea of the independence of science may appear. We may argue that psychiatry (or perhaps more broadly, medical science) is a form of 'socio-intellectual force'. That is to say, it represents an approach that has aspects both of a social kind and of an intellectual kind. We can say that psychiatrists represent a social force because they gather together, speak to one another, share ideas, and so forth. They also have organizations that represent their interests as a professional group, and so forth. However, they also represent an intellectual force. That is to say, they represent a particular kind of approach to problems such as those of children or adults with ADHD. This intellectual force lies in the power of scientific approach, the ideas, and theorizations of medicine, and the technologies that seek out or suggest evidence for them.

In this sense, the diagnosis of ADHD and indeed the very idea of ADHD represents not a political intellectual force (individualization) but a conceptual intellectual force (medicalization, if you like). To unmask ADHD, in the light of its intellectual or conceptual commitments, is to do no more than to say that ADHD is a scientific idea. And this is in no way to damage it as an idea. Far from rendering it practically ineffective, all this does is to identify the kind of approach that ADHD represents in its own terms.

And this is what I have been arguing for over the last two chapters in answer to the sceptic. The sceptic thinks that mental illness or specific mental illness diagnoses such as ADHD represent something other than a medical response to behavioural issues. To support this, we have seen how two potentially sceptical approaches might seek to argue for the existence or reality of this non-medical response. But neither has succeeded. The strong programme in the sociology of knowledge sought to show that mental illness was a reproduction of a social exclusion of some form. But it tripped up over the idea of reproduction. The sceptical social constructionist, as we have seen in this chapter, seeks to show that ADHD is an individualization of a social problem and so to unmask it. But it does not allow for the possibility that to individualize a problem might represent something other than a political environment or force. I have argued that in fact it represents a medical conceptualization or force.

It could be said, at this point, that all I have done is to say, in effect, that ADHD is medicalization. And, it could reasonably be pointed out, this is not much of an achievement. Worse, it is precisely the accusation levelled at psychiatry by sceptics. However, this is to miss the force of my point. Medicalization is usually taken to mean the application of medical ideas in places where they are not appropriate. But there is a neutral sense of the term. ADHD—and indeed mental illness in general—seem to me to be a place where this neutral use of the term medicalize is correct. It refers to an approach to an area that may well be controversial. In the case of ADHD it certainly seems to me that it is. And the radical questions and sceptical answers that have been the main theme of this book have aimed to suggest that what is true of ADHD is true of other mental illnesses too, and of mental illness in general. The idea of illness in the areas where we have identified it—in the realm of beliefs, ideas, values, behaviours, and so on—certainly is controversial or capable of being made controversial. But it is not necessarily, or by that token, wrong.

The metaphor of mental illness—or specific metaphors such as ADHD—reflect a certain kind of interest or approach being taken in human affairs. That interest is not necessarily to be understood as in the service of something else—a political or any other form of agenda or commitment. That is not to say that it cannot be argued that it is: but it is to say that such arguments will need to go beyond the sorts of arguments looked at in this chapter and the last.

Endnote

1 In making all these and subsequent claims, I have been immensely aided by Ian Hacking's no-nonsense book The Social Construction of What? (Hacking, 1999).

8 Metaphors and models

8.1 Introduction

In the previous two chapters of this part of the book I have wanted to hold on to the idea that someone may remake the world by using metaphor, without falling into scepticism about mental illness or particular mental illnesses such as ADHD.

What I suggested was that science, in so far as it makes the world, makes it in causal, physical, structural, or functional terms. Such terms, if not peculiar to natural or medical science, are at least that sort of descriptive term that scientists such as psychiatrists seek. Unless the psychiatrist also makes the social world in terms of this kind, then the social world will be made in one way and the phenomena that the psychiatrist investigates will be made in a different way. From this I concluded that mental illnesses cannot represent reproductions of social attitudes, and that while mental illnesses may be constructions, they are not social constructions. So, psychiatry, even if it does involve our recategorization of the world, does not necessarily involve doing so simply in line with our social, religious, political, or ethical attitudes.

However, even if I can hold the line on these matters, I still seem to have a problem that I identified earlier. Metaphor is unruly. It does not submit to the existing boundaries of classification or conceptualization, but on the contrary seeks to exceed or break them. It seems to this extent to be irrational, or at any rate non-rational. The problem is this: I seem to have introduced this unruly element into science, and this seems to threaten its rationality.

Someone may say that this problem, and others I have previously been seeking to avoid, could have been eluded altogether. If I did not hold that metaphors actually change how the world is, by changing how we think of it and what we may perceive in it, I would have an easier time. Suppose I did not hold that mental illness was made a reality of the world, or more accurately has the kind of reality it has, in virtue of the use of metaphors such as schizophrenia is an illness. Then I would not need to worry that metaphors might represent an attempt to impose a social belief upon people. Nor would it then matter in quite the same way if metaphor is an unruly, non-rational thing.

Moreover, this is not an idle speculation: alternative ways of thinking of metaphor are available. One is that we might think of metaphor as a piece of advice. It suggests we try something out: Had you tried thinking of it this way? Advice does not so much seek to change how things are or even how they appear to be, but to provide a fruitful mode of thought. If I saw metaphors as advisory, I could accept that metaphors might come from social beliefs and interests, because they would not then be making or remaking the world. They would not represent any kind of imposition on the world, and nor would they be deceptive. Alternatively, I could take up the idea that metaphors are what Richard Rorty (1991) calls unfamiliar noises. This is an idea that is part of Rorty's pragmatist agenda, in that, among other things, he seeks to replace—or redefine—concern with the truth about how things are with what he calls solidarity—that is to say, in broad terms, an agreement about what represents the best way for our society (the one we are actually part of and committed to) to handle some issue or problem.

Furthermore, the concern for science's rationality would also be unwarranted, or at least less urgent. Szasz thinks that metaphor is unmanageable and unruly, which seems to lend weight to his cautions against sciences, such as psychiatry, which are based upon it. Such sciences, Szasz claims, do not have objective features of the world to concentrate on. They create their own realities. They do not have to, indeed logically they cannot, match themselves up against these. Metaphors, as we characteristically see them in the hands of poets, are not to be tested or experimented upon. They are not presented in poems as verifiable, confirmable, or even falsifiable comments about how things are. Szasz suggests that in the hands of scientists, similar latitude cannot be allowed.

However, if metaphors are advisory, or are to be understood as unfamiliar noises that may suddenly open up a new avenue in the search for the best way ahead for our community, then they can be accepted or rejected without getting involved in an argument about whether these things really exist or not. If metaphors make suggestions rather than definite propositions, or try to surprise us into better ways of dealing with something, then a decent degree of rationality seems to be preserved in science, while some of the advantages of the radical and unexpected concerning how one might think of things are preserved too.

Notwithstanding the advantages that may seem to flow from thinking of metaphor in these ways, I shall not take up the idea that they must play this kind of role. They may do; my purpose is not to rule it out. However, I do not think that the notion of mental illness, or that the body is a machine, or that schizophrenia or ADHD are illnesses need to be, or are most plausibly construed either as advisory or in the pragmatist spirit of Rorty. This chapter will take these issues up.

But having rejected the idea that these metaphors are advisory, or to be understood in the pragmatist's terms, the issue of irrationality returns. The answer to the worry that the presence of metaphor as I describe it throws science into unreason or irrationality is, to some degree, simply to accept it. The worry has to be lived with. However, a rational process that relies upon metaphor can be discerned. From the recategorization of the mad as ill created by metaphor may arise models of particular aspects of madness. A model is fundamentally an attempted analogy, as in the example of a musical instrument as a model for the human vocal organs in *Gray's Anatomy* (see Chapter 5). Models are intended to be testable. They are produced by scientists to aid explanation and understanding, and they can be rejected if they do not. The scientist pitches her ideas against her own beliefs about the world in the form of theories, hypotheses, and models. This is a rational process. What leaves the charge of unreason untouched is this belief: metaphors cannot be tested. Metaphors, rather than being the subject of tests, make tests possible. Indeed, this is one of metaphor's principal roles within science.

8.2 Advice and metaphor

Metaphors as advices

I will turn first to the idea that metaphor could be regarded as advisory.

Gray's Anatomy states that we should think of the human body 'as a complex of machinery'. The *Journal of Mental Health* suggests that 'insanity is purely a disease of the brain'. Psychiatrists think that schizophrenia is an illness or that some children and adults who have difficulty attending when they should have ADHD. I have taken all these to be examples of metaphor. They can be construed as recategorizations of the phenomena in question.

One has to be slightly careful how one puts this point. I do not want to give the impression that insanity and mental illness are necessarily simply terms for the same thing. This might suggest that we could specify some other classification that applies to the phenomena, and that refers to what first insanity and later brain disease refer to. Nor, analogously, do I think that ADHD necessarily refers to the same thing as say hyperkinesis or emotional disturbance or any of the other names that are sometimes said to have been bestowed on ADHD behaviours. This is not how I think it is, certainly not how it has to be.

Rather, recategorization may actually lead to different divisions among phenomena, and, indeed, to different phenomena. What counted as insanity in the eighteenth century may consist of a different range of phenomena to what comes to count as brain disease or as mental illness in the nineteenth and twentieth centuries. Allowing for this, I have taken the phrasing of these metaphors literally: that is to say I have seen them as expressing the idea that the body *is* a machine, or that madness *is* a brain disease, or that schizophrenia *is* an illness.

However, each could be taken in an advisory way. Rather than representing a recategorization, they could be taken to represent potentially useful or fruitful ways of conceptualizing the body, insanity, and schizophrenia respectively. They may say not 'the body is a machine', but 'try thinking of the body as if it were a machine'; not that 'insanity is a disease of the brain', but 'try thinking of insanity as if it were a disease of the brain, and see what arises'. The long-term survival of these pieces of advice would then be put down to the fact that they have proved fertile indeed. From 'try thinking of the body as if it were a piece of mechanism' all sorts of specific machine analogies have arisen that have proved useful in teaching, understanding, and treatment. *Gray's* fruitfully takes up the idea that the human vocal organs can be understood as a kind of machine. In what appears to be the same spirit, Engelhardt (1984) suggests that 'characterizations of clinical problems are ways in which one transforms ill-structured problems into problems with a structure *useful* with regard to offering predictions and other therapeutic interventions' (p. 34; my italics).

The utility of such pieces of advice may be restricted. It may be advice that works in only some cases and only for some purposes. If an explanation of how the lungs inhale air is sought, then the analogy with bellows may be to the point; but if we want to know how they absorb oxygen from the air, the model or analogy of bellows is no longer helpful. Some other mechanical analogy may be needed, or we may need to try a different kind of analogy all together. The mechanical is but one way or level of looking at the body. However, the body could usefully be thought to be like or modelled on several other things. Henrik Wulff, for example, considers a number of models of man that might be appealed to in medicine (Wulff, 1994). The functioning structure model is only one of these, and, says Wulff, a fairly basic one at that.

On this account, in the area of psychiatry, the claim that insanity is a disease of the brain would become a suggestion. 'Try thinking of it in these terms. If you do, that may lead to all sorts of advantages of understanding and management.' This piece of advice might be combined with others. A Wulffian variety of useful models might be generated: one condition may be thought of in neurological terms, another in functional, and another in more behavioural terms, and so forth. At no point need schizophrenia be completely identified with physical disease. Indeed, we could abandon the question what kind of thing mental illness really is. Insanity could be a brain disease for some purposes and not for others.

And metaphors may be particularly good at generating this sort of advice. They can bring all sorts of things together for advisory purposes, perhaps generating a rich variety of equally rich analogies.

Advice and the logical positivists

I derive the idea that some statements in science may be advisory from the work of Alan Ryan (1970). Ryan contrasts these advisory statements with the two kinds allowed by the logical positivists, a group of writers who worked in Vienna in the 1920 and 30s (cf. Hanfling, 1981, pp. 1–4), and whose views were memorably propounded in English by A.J. Ayer in his book *Language, Truth and Logic* (1978; first published in 1936). It is worth glancing briefly at Ryan's argument, because, although he does not speak of metaphor, and it is far from clear he would agree with the claims we have been making, it is relevant to our understanding of the role of metaphor.

The logical positivists held that only those statements of fact whose truth or falsity can in principle be verified make any sense, and that only statements that make sense can be candidates for factual knowledge (Ayer, 1978, pp. 48–9; Chalmers, 1982, p. xviii). Another group of propositions also makes sense; these are tautologies. And they make sense because of the meanings of their words (see Ayer, 1978, particularly chapter 4). The logical positivists, or at any rate Ayer, thought that only statements that are tautologies or are observation statements (or are based upon these) made sense. Tautologies are like statements we considered earlier that are true (or false) by definition: 'a triangle has four sides' is false by definition; 'a straight line is the shortest distance between two points' true by definition (at least in Euclidean geometry). Observation statements, or statements based upon observations, are like another set of statements we considered earlier. 'There are planets around other stars': 'there is no natural earth satellite apart from the moon'. The truth of these statements is established or refuted on the basis of our observations. The logical positivists ruled all statements senseless, and hence useless to science or anything else, which were not either tautologies or observations or based upon them.

Ryan thinks that the logical positivists have missed something. He argues that advisory statements do have a role in science, despite failing to make sense on logical positivist criteria. To take an example: *think of the body as a machine*. This is not tautological: it is not like $2 \times 5 = 10$ or triangles have three sides, statements that are, according to the logical positivists, true by definition. It does not tell you the meanings of words. It is a suggestion. Nor is it based on observation: it is not a factual generalization such as 'the sun rises everyday' that is based upon the observation that it rose today, yesterday, and the day before. Instead it suggests something we might try out. Saying the body is a machine suggests a way of thinking about the body.

Someone might counter that ways of thinking in science should follow on from observations or things detected by technical means. So, we should start thinking of the body as a machine only after we have observed its machine-like properties: our advice should be based upon good experience. This seems reasonable for some cases. Some pieces of advice in science may be thought of as connected to certain discoveries, in the sense that certain discoveries may have led people to think in these terms. Plausibly, discoveries about vibrations in the air and sound led people to think of the human vocal organs in terms of resonators and columns of air, and this in turn leads to the idea that they can be modelled upon a musical instrument.

However, advisory suggestions which may be based upon observations do not by any means exhaust the category. Ryan's principal example makes it clear that he does not think of advice being dependent upon observation. He illustrates advisory ways of thinking with Kant's notion that space was Euclidean. That is to say it was describable in terms of Euclid's geometry in that, for example, a straight line is the shortest distance between two points, and there are only three physical dimensions. This is certainly how it appears to observation. Ryan says Kant thought this was a necessary truth about space. However, Kant's confidence in the necessity of Euclidean space in human knowledge was premature. It was clear 'by the time relativistic physics was established that this [Kant's] belief . . . made for grave difficulties when applied to the calculations involved in stellar mechanics—and so another geometry was adopted' (Ryan, 1970, p. 68). In retrospect, Kant's view of what space must be turned out to be only one of a number of possibilities; something it could be thought of as being but did not have to be. Kant's idea that space is necessarily Euclidean can be reconstructed as a piece of advice. In the long run, at least on the stellar level, this did not prove to be the best piece of advice. However, it is difficult to see how this piece of advice to think of space as having more than three dimensions could be based on observation.

Euclidean geometry was abandoned at stellar levels because it was not fruitful to try to work with it there any more and not because observation suggested an alternative. The notion of fruitfulness is not to be run together with the notions of true and false, or right and wrong. Ryan suggests that advice is not to be judged for its verifiability by observation or logical analysis, the two alternatives offered by logical positivism (Ryan, 1970, p. 67). Fruitfulness will be judged by other criteria. Perhaps it enables the doing of things, or opens up new theories or lines of questioning. Once we think of the body as if it were a machine we can think of all sorts of machines that particular parts of the body may be like; bellows, computers, musical instruments. At any rate, statements of the advisory kind seem to be a part of science, without being verifiable; fruitful within the scientific endeavour without being true or false.

Ryan's account seems to me perfectly plausible for some statements. Perhaps those about space. And I would not like to rule out the possibility that metaphor can be used in this advisory way. Four dimensional space might be regarded as a metaphor. Moreover, Ryan's analysis of how advisory statements fall outside the categories allowed by logical positivism is one that applies to my account of metaphor too. Metaphors, whether advisory or classificatory have a legitimate role in science but appear not to be tautological or observational. Metaphor as I have spoken of it falls into a category that is at any rate extremely awkward to fit in with either of these. As the Pasteur case shows, metaphors have a role in science, but are not based on observation. They may create rather than record the features of things. However, to describe them as tautological is somewhat awkward too. In the Pasteur case, we do not seem to have a tautology for the simple reason that Pasteur's use of the term vaccination is, if anything, a mistake in the circumstances. In either case, from the logical positivist view, we have an error needing correction. The logical positivist cannot make room for the idea of advice or for the idea of reclassificatory metaphor.

But why do I not settle for the idea that metaphors represent a piece of advice, and are to be judged upon their fruitfulness?

The reason will become clearer in the section after next, where I will look at the relation between metaphors and models. Models are plausibly advisory. We can shift from one model to another as we attempt to understand or explain something. But what we will find is that metaphor lies behind models, representing an entrenched view of how the world is to be categorized. It is correct to speak of these entrenched metaphors as creative or classificatory rather than advisory; they play a part in making the world what it is. They go beyond giving advice about how we may look at it for certain purposes. They appear to be given in the world, taking the form of natural existences and boundaries. This is something about which the strong programme in the sociology of knowledge seems to me to be correct, and it is also reflected in social constructionist approach to such ideas as ADHD. It is, in the case of mental illness or ADHD, the metaphor that makes possible certain kinds of advice, or of models that may be created to aid the investigation of such conditions.

8.3 A pragmatist account of metaphor

In the next section, then, I shall argue that a metaphor may come to express a more or less entrenched view of how things are: 'insanity is a disease of the brain', 'the combination of inattentive, hyperactive and impulsive behaviours is ADHD'. For this reason, I shall hold that metaphors play a part in making some aspects of the world: they are not just advices or suggestions. But before I argue that, I shall take a look at a view of things, put forward by pragmatists such as Richard Rorty (1980, 1991, 1995), which seeks to remove from our thought concerns about how things really are, and replace it with something very different. Rorty is a particularly important figure for my purposes, because he offers a notion of metaphor that, arguably, sees the imagination of the poet taking a central role in science. To this extent, my ideas are rather like his. But he connects this to an approach to the idea that mental illness, or particular mental illnesses, are real that seeks to re-evaluate what that idea might mean. In short, he takes a radical look at some of the radical questions with which I started this book.

In this section I shall focus initially upon this re-evaluation of those radical questions, in the context of which Rorty develops his ideas about metaphor. I shall not be able to do Rorty's overarching view justice, of course. But as it has a number of parallels (and some differences) with the one I have advanced in this book, it will be useful to say something about Rorty's larger picture here. I shall gradually focus in upon his idea of metaphor.

The radical question I asked, using Szasz's words, right at the beginning of the book was: does mental illness exist? I have argued that it does—but the way in that it exists is perhaps not one that most who consider Szasz's question would have expected or would accept. It exists, I have argued, as a human idea—produced through a categorizing metaphor. Through this metaphor a particular kind of approach—the medical approach—pursues and interprets evidence of illness in a variety of conditions. In this sense, and in this way, human agency creates mental illnesses.

What might a pragmatic approach say about the radical question Szasz posed? And what might it say about my answer? The question at first sight appears to be about whether there is something in nature—something that medical science could study and understand—called mental illness. Or, if we take some of the specific radical questions such as Boyle's question about schizophrenia or Breggin's about ADHD, these questions appear to be about whether these things exist. Is there any such thing in existence that has the nature of schizophrenia or ADHD? (And when we look at the nature of these things—when we look at the kind of things they are said to be by those who do believe in them—we find this means that they are claimed to exist as illnesses.) Because such questions appear to ask about something in nature, it can be argued that these questions look very like the ones someone would ask if she thought that 'the goal of scientific enquiry into man is to understand "underlying structures," or "culturally invariant factors," or "biologically determined patterns"' (Rorty, 1991, p. 22).

Rorty takes it that the search for all these—underlying structures and so on—represents the belief in a reference point for truths, which is conceived as being outside any particular community. In the sort of terms in that Latour talks about the dualism of the moderns, we might say that these things are thought to come from the hand of nature: they are not the products of people or communities. Rorty seems to be speaking in a similar vein when he says they are conceived as parts of a non-human reality (p. 21). Rorty says that it is supposed, by those who seek after these structures, or at least believe that truth is referenced to them, that to find out about these one must come into some form of direct contact with them. The model of this access in the modern world has been, Rorty believes, the 'Newtonian physical scientist' (p. 22). This individual has an ability to pierce through appearance to reality and to arrive at knowledge rather than opinion (p. 22). In contrast, any approach that goes via surface features, culturally determined factors, or socially determined patterns will fail because it sets up some form of veil between itself and the object of study.

Rorty thinks that these attitudes, and in particular the search for truth referenced to something outside our communities, reflects one way in which, historically, people have sought to respond to one of the fundamental issues humankind faces, namely how to give sense and meaning to their lives. Giving meaning to one's life, Rorty suggests, involves finding a larger context into which to fit one's existence. Rorty notes that something conceived to be outside any particular community certainly seems to meet this need for meaning. However, he also thinks that seeking to find some reference point that transcends one's own community is not the only way in which to achieve this sense of meaning. His large project, which he calls pragmatism, aims to suggest another way to find meaning.

He wants to replace the reference point of something outside any and all real communities with a reference point within a particular community (or perhaps a number of reference points within particular communities). He aims to replace the itch to find objectivity with the desire for solidarity in the pursuit of the betterment of things within and by the lights of one's own community. Rorty's approach is, then, as he readily admits, ethnocentric: it does not seek something that transcends particular communities. But, he argues, in fact we have no choice but to be ethnocentric: the dream of making contact with something that transcends our communities is a hopeless dream. He argues that truth, as usually conceived, represents this dream.

However, the fact that humans have nothing to cling to other than notions of what is best generated within real communities, does not mean we in our community have to be closed to alternatives, or be dogmatic or jingoistic about the standards we set. Solidarity, in the eyes of the community to which Rorty pledges allegiance (that is to say the modern, Western Liberal democratic community), is represented by the idea of 'unforced agreement' (p. 38). This in turn represents the difference, in a pragmatic sense, between the rational and the irrational (p. 48). The rational, in the pragmatic sense, is related to persuasion—to reasonableness (p. 37) (which includes openness, tolerance, and other liberal virtues). In contrast, forced agreement is the paradigm of unreasonableness. Rorty notes that science is usually represented as our most rational means in the pursuit of truth. However, for the pragmatist, Rorty argues, science represents reasonableness. That is to say, at least as an ideal, it is a community of open tolerant people. Rorty admits that in reality science may not achieve this, but is none the less our best model of it.

This, then, is Rorty's general approach, not too badly damaged by the way I have packaged it, I hope. How far does it fit in with my views and how far are they in tension with one another? One area where both similarities and differences emerge is between my treatment of the likeness argument and Rorty's criticism of traditional ideas of rationality. Rorty says that the non-pragmatic—the traditional, truth oriented—approach to rationality is to specify in advance what will count as success. He gives several examples of the traditional rationality he has in mind:

> [W]e think of judges as knowing in advance what criteria a brief will have to satisfy in order to invoke a favorable decision, and of business people as setting well-defined goals and being judged by their success in achieving them. Law and business are good examples of rationality, but the scientist, knowing in advance what would count as disconfirming his hypothesis and prepared to abandon that hypothesis as the result of the unfavorable outcome of a single experiment, seems a truly heroic example. Further, we seem to have a clear criterion for the success of a scientific theory—namely, its ability to predict, and thereby enable us to control some portion of the world. (p. 36)

We can convert this to a story of someone looking for an answer to Szasz's radical question about mental illness, or Breggin's radical question about

ADHD. The story we might generate is of someone who would take a prior notion of what mental illness was, or of what would make something an illness, and then set out to discover whether or not ADHD fits that description. Such a person, the rational story says, should be willing to give up the idea that ADHD is an illness if it is discovered not to have the features known to make things illnesses. This mirrors the approach of the likeness argument. The likeness argument starts with a notion of what illness is like—what its defining features are—and then goes out to find if putative mental illnesses have those features.

Rorty wants to replace this traditional idea of the rational approach with something very different. It would be something more like an agreement that, by the lights of our society, the best way of dealing with those who present us with certain sorts of difficulty, is to treat them as ill. This, it might be argued, is the best way forward we can come up with in the case of those who have problems with thoughts in their heads they say are not theirs, or who drink too much, or cannot concentrate on their school work. In our community, then, the medical approach to such problems seems to be the best. For example, it might appear to be the approach that seems most humanitarian—which for example treats these people as needing help, rather than being blamed. Or it might be said to represent the value that we place on the individual. Such beliefs about the best way to approach the behaviours in question do not rely on the sort of rationality that the likeness argument appears to express: they do not represent claims about what sort of thing ADHD really is, for example.

The most obvious parallel between Rorty's approach and mine arises from the fact that I hold that the likeness argument is mistaken in thinking that the features of things decide what category they should be placed in. The features of things do not determine that. Rather, humans place things into categories, and in the light of that, certain sorts of features appear. That is to say we cannot say in advance what might decide whether (say) we should regard schizophrenia as an illness or not. The metaphors by which schizophrenia or ADHD become illnesses, or by which madness (in general) becomes mental illness, arise in the imagination of scientists, or perhaps wider society, but not through any rational procedure based upon observation, for example. It could be that the metaphor of illness suggests itself for reasons that are to do with what modern society regards as the humane approach. So my point of quarrel with the likeness argument might fit in with Rorty's pragmatism.

However, I think there may also be a point of tension between my ideas and Rorty's pragmatic approach. It arises in the claim, which I made for example in the last chapter on ADHD, that to categorize something as ADHD is to bring to it a description of a medical form. I described this as having, broadly, two aspects: a psychological characteristic and a causally associated brain abnormality. These I characterized as entailing the individualization of the problem—that is to say, the location of the problem within the individual person rather than in his or her context. Moreover, I have noted on several occasions that medical explanations generally take the form of functional or causal accounts, and are couched in the language of biology, or whatever other science might be involved. They involve relations between materials of the kind that these sciences generally work with, for example. All this, in one way and another, could be said to come with the metaphor. It is inherent in categorizing something as an illness that these descriptive resources become applicable.

So what appears to have happened is that I have fixed the meaning of a term such as illness. It appears that I argue that when something is categorized, it acquires a preordained set of features. This would happen through the metaphor. This would mean that the metaphor would be more than simply a categorization—it would impose a specific set of features on the condition.

This would put Rorty's account and mine somewhat at odds. However, I shall suggest that this appearance is false. Beyond that, I will suggest that Rorty's account has a problem that my approach does not have.

Rorty would not, I think, accept that metaphor represents the application of a pre-existing meaning. This is despite the fact that like Davidson he believes that the words in metaphors retain their ordinary common-or-garden senses. If phrases such as ADHD is an illness, insanity is a disease of the brain and mental illness are metaphors, Rorty would argue, they mean just what they say. The words illness and disease in these phrases do not have a special meaning—for example, a secondary sense (Gipps, 2003, and see Chapter 4) or a meaning particular to the mental (Svensson, 1980, and see Chapter 4). However, this is not because Davidson or Rorty think that metaphors simply leave everything as it was. Rather, Davidson and Rorty have a causal account of how metaphors work. The meanings of the words are, at least as far as the consequence of using metaphor goes, somewhat otiose. This is because, Rorty and Davidson both think that 'that semantical notions like "meaning" have a role only within the quite narrow . . . limits of regular, predictable, linguistic behaviour—the limits which mark off (temporarily) the literal use of language' (Rorty, 1991, pp. 163–4). They believe that metaphor works outside these predictable, regular limits of linguistic behaviour. It is not, we might say, subject to the traditional idea of rationality.

To explain their views of how metaphor works, both Rorty and Davidson use some memorable images. Rorty calls metaphor an 'unfamiliar noise'—an unexpected linguistic event if you like. Davidson calls it the 'dream-work of language' and compares it with having a bang on the head. Both think metaphor is an unusual or unexpected event in the world around us. As a result of the metaphorical bang on the head that metaphor gives one, Davidson suggests one might have pictures in the mind. And pictures, Davidson notes, are pictures, not new propositions or ideas expressed in the ordinary meanings of words. Hearing the metaphor 'light wave' the physicist perhaps has visions of superimposed bright objects and ocean waves. How the scientist's thought might then go on is not predictable from this picture. Applying this to a metaphor I suggested earlier (the body is a machine) might give the medical scientist images of clocks, pumps, car engines and so forth juxtaposed with images of human bodies (the specific machines imagined will be historically contingent). And hearing the metaphor ADHD is an illness the psychiatrist may have images of children failing to meet the expectations of their teachers and hopes of their parents and being out of control in some way, alongside images of people with colds, measles, and other diseases.

However, different to this, I seem to be saying that to conceptualize ADHD behaviours in terms of ADHD is to conceptualize them in the sort of terms science, medicine, and psychiatry already make use of. I seem to rely on the ordinary meanings of words in metaphor. So this seems to mean I would certainly find myself in disagreement with Rorty on this particular point.

But Rorty cannot simply leave his explanation at this point: Rorty claims that a metaphor can become a proposition or a statement (insanity is a disease of the brain). It is difficult to see how this could be true of unexpected events in general. The survival of Pasteur's chickens was an unexpected event, as we have seen. But it is not something that conveys any cognitive content. Nor are Rorty's own examples, such as coming across an anomalous creature such as a Platypus or object such as a Pulsar (1991, p. 167). The difference that Rorty acknowledges between these unexpected events and objects and metaphors, is that metaphors may become linguistic behaviours. This is what happens when they die into literalness, as he puts it (1991, p. 167). When metaphors become dead, he claims, and become part of the predictable manageable linguistic behaviour of the community, they begin to convey information, and to act as justifications for belief (cf. pp. 170–2). However, there is a problem in seeing what this 'dying off into literalness' comes to. How does an unexpected noise acquire the status of a statement?

So Rorty has a difficulty here, but I will not try to resolve it on his behalf. On the other hand, for me, because I think that metaphors can be categorizations, they are more than unfamiliar noises or unexpected events. They express something, so there is not so much of a puzzle about how they get converted into more ordinary, expected, noises. They do express something—a thought or idea. And this also allows for the possibility that they might come to be regarded as something unexpected again. Categorizations can be changed more than once. The metaphor ADHD is an illness or insanity is a disease of the brain can come to seem perfectly ordinary and obvious non-metaphors for a time, and then be questioned and doubted, so that their metaphorical nature is reasserted.

So, on this particular issue, I disagree with Rorty. However, I do not think this means that I hold that metaphor is the application of a fixed definable and immutable meaning. And here I think my account is close again to Rorty's, at least in spirit, if not in detail. I do not think that categorizing something as an illness decides what features it shall have in any conceptually fixed way. What I want to argue in the next section is that the features that categorizing conditions such as schizophrenia as illnesses gives rise to, are decided in terms of models that the categorizing makes possible. This means that we cannot say in advance what particular features say schizophrenia may be said to have. Medicine has a history and is always developing. What features schizophrenia may have will depend on what models have been developed. All we can say, in the light of the categorization of schizophrenia or ADHD or alcoholism as illnesses, is that they will be models that reflect that categorization.

8.4 Metaphors and models

Some models in medicine

In 1628 in *de Motu Cordis* William Harvey suggested that the heart pumps the blood around an enclosed circulatory system (Harvey, 1928). At the time Harvey made his suggestion only the large blood carrying vessels the arteries and veins were known to exist. There was no known connection between these two kinds of vessel. In suggesting that the system involved circulation, Harvey had to hypothesize that there were vessels, too small to be observed, which completed the system, allowing the blood to flow out from and back to the heart. These vessels, the capillaries, were discovered later in the century after his death when microscope power and technique achieved the means to view them. In this respect, Harvey's hypothesis was tested and proved robust (see Harré, 1985, p. 93; Bynum and Porter, 1997, p. 122; Clendening, 1960, pp. 152–69, 209–13, for some account of these events and further sources).

Harvey's hypothesis arises from a particular picture of human circulation. This picture we can call a model; or we can say that Harvey modelled the flow of blood in the human on this picture. Had the capillaries never been found, but some other mechanism altogether identified, Harvey's hypothesis, and with it his picture and his model, would have been tested and found wanting. Likewise, with *Gray's* musical instrument model of the human vocal organs; that too could have been, and may yet be, found wanting.

Within psychiatric medicine similar modelling can be found. A good nineteenth century example is Pierre Falret's use of the physical disease progressive paralysis to model *folie circulaire* (manic-depressive illness) as a single illness, which expressed itself first in one way and then in another (see Lanczik and Beckman, 1991, pp. 6–7). Another example is of paediatrician George Still, who became interested in problem behaviours in children. Right from the start he suggested that the correct model for understanding children with what might now be called conduct disorder, oppositional defiant disorder, and ADHD was that of brain impairment. While the children with various conduct problems did not show brain lesions, Still believed the model was the correct one. He hypothesized that the brain lesions would one day show up (Still, 1902). One other author whose work featured as an example of a likeness argument earlier is clearly an example too of the use of a model. Claridge tries to persuade us that the correct model for schizophrenia is to be found in systemic diseases such as hypertension (Claridge, 1992). Claridge's assumption is that we can model it on some sort of disease or other (and in this also lies the assumption of the likeness argument).

Claridge seeks to support his model and perhaps to demonstrate its fruitfulness by referring to further evidence that suggests that schizophrenia, like hypertension, has a genetic basis: '[T]here is now good evidence (Kety 1985) that schizotypal disorder and schizophrenia are genetically related, suggesting that the former is a partial expression of similar underlying traits. . . . What is most likely . . . is that it is the dispositional aspects that are inherited, as is true of many other human traits.' (Kety, 1985; Claridge, 1992, p. 165).

Claridge is using the features of his model (hypertension) to propose that there will be genetic connections in schizophrenia; his model fruitfully suggests this further possibility. He refers to the work of Kety to provide support for his proposal. He also uses features of hypertension to suggest that it would be apposite to look for less obvious examples of schizophrenia than those usually seen by psychiatrists: 'One feature [of the model] that deserves further comment is the assumption, based on the parallel drawn here with the physical systemic disease, that mild or subclinical varieties of schizophrenia can occur.' (1992, p. 164).

Claridge does indeed direct us towards what he regards as evidence that such subclinical varieties of schizophrenia do occur (Kety, 1985). Again, he tries to use his model to expand the ways in which schizophrenia is understood and thought about.

Models, metaphors, and tests

One shared feature of the various models we have considered is the idea that they can be pitched against the scientist's beliefs about the world. Models such as those proposed by Harvey, Still, and Claridge can be tested. Claridge's reference to Kety is a sort of test. If Claridge's suggestion that schizophrenia be modelled upon hypertension were either true or at least fertile, further likenesses could be expected to appear. Kety is said to have identified a subclinical variety of schizophrenia, something that we find also in hypertension. Perhaps if the notion that we are genetically disposed to schizophrenia (as we are said to be to hypertension) were taken up in a research programme, then some evidence would emerge that would appear either to lend support to his view or to undermine it. Stories of the development of the medical understanding of ADHD often aim to show how gradually evidence of the existence of the brain abnormalities Still guessed were there was gathered. The advent of brain imaging devices (e.g. PET scanners) is usually seen as the latest chapter in this gradual working out of Still's ideas. The existence or absence of genetic correlations, abnormalities in particular brain areas, or physiological abnormalities that may be observed in PET scanners and the like, serve as the sort of evidence to which models have to answer. If they fail such tests they need to be adjusted or abandoned.

All these features of Claridge's model can be comfortably accommodated by sceptical arguments, though of course with the purpose of showing that medical models of schizophrenia are mere verbal acrobatics. Szasz, for example, claims that an extended metaphor can become a model. That is to say that once one term has illicitly crossed from its proper place of use into an area where it has no business, a whole range of other associated words may follow together with the relations and connections they imply. The word illness becomes improperly associated with schizophrenia, and before we know it, the whole gamut of medical terms turns up and starts associating with it too. From a single point of metaphorical contact, the entire medical model of things arrives to shape schizophrenia's future. The medical picture of schizophrenia perhaps develops through the figurative comparisons mentioned by Tirrell (see Chapter 4). What Szasz would probably say is going on with Claridge's argument is this: it presents us with yet another opportunity to speak in terms associated with illness about something (human behaviour) that can be disordered, diseased, or ill only metaphorically. Claridge argues that as we can have subclinical hypertension, we can expect to find subclinical schizophrenia. However, for Szasz the word subclinical, applied to human behaviours, would be metaphorical. For him there can no more be subclinical behaviours than there can be clinical behaviours.

As has been the case previously, I tend to agree with what I take it the thrust of the sceptical analysis would be without thereby reaching its sceptical conclusion. The central point of agreement between myself and a sceptic in Claridge's case would be this: Claridge is indeed extending a metaphor. Underlying, and making possible Claridge's modelling of schizophrenia upon hypertension is the idea that schizophrenia is an illness. The model Claridge uses simply assumes that schizophrenia is an illness of some kind. That is to say it presumes the presence of phenomena that will be explicable in the form of some illness model. A sceptic such as Szasz would be right to see the metaphor he objects to in the very heart of the model that Claridge advances.

If we look at Claridge's reasoning in a little more detail we can see the presumption emerging in the circularity of his reasoning. Even though he suggests that genes underlie only a disposition to schizophrenia, his whole argument assumes that this disposition should be seen in illness terms. This circularity cannot be avoided, and it appears as an arbitrary element in his reasoning. Claridge seems to have the idea that 'many other human traits' are to be included in the same analysis. He may have in mind other traits or dispositions to illness. If so, that also reveals the circularity of his position. That is it reveals his assumption that schizophrenia is an illness and will be explicable in illness terms. But he may be thinking rather of non-pathological behaviours: perhaps he thinks we are genetically disposed to be nervous, or to act kindly. However, if we take this suggestion seriously, then the existence of the genetic disposition to schizophrenia does not add any weight to the claim that this is a particularly interesting similarity to hypertension. In hypertension the genetic disposition is presumably accorded a causal role. However, it is far from clear that genetic dispositions related to behaviours have to be regarded causally, as our earlier arguments concerning alcoholism and ADHD sought to show.

Perhaps Claridge thinks that some non-pathological human behaviours do have a causal genetic dispositional aspect. He may think that the human trait for kindness is inherited. But if he does, then the analogy between schizophrenia and hypertension as an illness still seems to be purely arbitrary. Only Claridge's interest steers us to it. We might have gone the other way and argued that schizophrenia should not be modelled on hypertension or any other disease, but rather should be understood as we understand our kindness or other behaviours. This implicit circularity should not, however, surprise us: Claridge's position provides the basis of a likeness argument and, on the strong view of the mistake in likeness arguments, there is always an aspect of the arbitrary in them. A likeness argument about the existence of mental illness or about its nature is bound to be circular. It purports to be based on likenesses. However, their existence actually depends on an assumption of the conclusion of the argument before it begins. And this makes any circular argument arbitrary in the sense that genuine support for its conclusions must lie somewhere outside it, in a domain the argument does not specify. Something other than the resources offered by his argument sustains Claridge's conclusion that schizophrenia is an illness of some kind.

Someone may say that as models such as that Claridge explores are derived from metaphors, any test of the model is a test of the metaphor upon which the model depends. In that case, the distinction proposed between metaphor and model evaporates. The scientist's metaphor ends up in the same court and before the same jury as his models.

To enlarge on this claim for a moment: consider again the model in *Gray's Anatomy* of the musical instrument for the human vocal organs.

> As in most musical instruments, the mechanism of speech consists of three essentials: a source of energy, structures capable of periodic and aperiodic oscillations and a resonator. Energy is derived from the velocity of the expired air, oscillation primarily from the vocal folds and resonance from the multiform 'column' of air extending from the folds to the lips and nostrils Williams *et al.* (1989, p. 1257)

Here, the description could, in principle, be countered. Perhaps the vocal organs are more like a musical instrument than they are like a bicycle pump. Equally, there may be some other machine that the vocal organs are even more akin to—for example, the voice box theoretical physicist Stephen Hawking uses. It is possible that a greater range of features of the vocal organs and their workings may be covered in one machine analogy than in another. It makes sense to question and test a specific analogy of machine to organ or system of the body. The claim we are considering is that questioning *which model* of the vocal organs is appropriate is equivalent to questioning the metaphor that makes the musical instrument model possible, in this case the metaphor the body is a machine.

However, there is no such equivalence. The metaphor makes possible not only the musical instrument model but also its rivals. We can, given that we think the body is a machine, assess various machine models, deciding which is the best. A challenge to the use of a specific machine analogy is one thing. It is quite another thing to question the identification of the body with the mechanical. I would claim that there is no way of questioning the identification of the body with the mechanical by means of any facts about the body. For the idea that the body is a piece of machinery is not based upon any of the facts about its parts. If the vocal organs are not much like a bicycle pump, nothing follows for the general identification of the body with machinery. By the same token, nothing much follows if the vocal organs are like another machine, a musical instrument for example.

To challenge the metaphor, that is, to challenge the idea that the body is a machine, is not to produce facts about the body, but to produce an alternative identification. It is to move the body from one category into another. In these circumstances, the idea that the vocal organs are like a musical instrument, in so far as the musical instrument is a machine, will indeed be rejected. However, this is because, if the alternative identification of the body is accepted, no facts about the body will seem to bear out any machine analogy for any part of the body any longer.

This is consistent with the strong view of the mistake in likeness arguments, in the case of schizophrenia in Claridge's argument, for example. The features that models model in the case of mental illness appear in virtue of the kind of thing we think it is. Genetic correlations appear as causal dispositions when internally related to the idea that schizophrenia is an illness of some sort. Given this, models based upon certain physical systemic diseases seem appropriate. Likewise, to refer back to our earlier arguments about alcoholism and ADHD, if we think that alcoholism or ADHD are illnesses then genetic correlations may well appear to be causal, and this feature may become a likeness between alcoholism and ADHD and other illnesses. However, neither the idea that alcoholism or ADHD are illnesses, nor by the same token, the metaphors expressed in the claims that alcoholism is an illness or that failures to pay attention in class are ADHD, depend on the features of likeness upon which specific models might be based: metaphors are not based upon features of things.

The conceptual point that lies behind these observations is that models depend upon metaphors, while metaphors do not depend upon models. This dependency takes the form that a model is an analogy appropriate to that range of features of or facts about some point or aspect of something (the body, schizophrenia, ADHD). This range of features or facts is itself made possible only in virtue of the kind of thing (a machine, an illness) that thing (the body, schizophrenia, ADHD) is thought to be.

Historical change of models

Historically, the appearance of models of a certain kind signals the category into that whatever it is they are models of has been placed. The appearance of mechanical models of aspects of the body (e.g. Harvey's of the circulation), or illness models of various kinds of madness (e.g. Falret's progressive paralysis model of *folie circulaire*), or of a behavioural pattern (e.g. the notion of defective moral self-control put forward by Still), suggests the recategorization of these. However, a change of models of a kind through time reflects a developing range of possibilities within a metaphor, rather than a change of metaphor. Machines change and develop, and the range of machine models will hence do so too. In the case of the brain, the modern notion of neural networks may replace the idea of the computer, as the computer analogy replaced those derived from more primitive machines. A series of different mechanical models of the workings of the human body may supersede one another through time, while the metaphor on which they are based is retained.

As machines develop, new machine analogies subvert older ones, replacing them. But metaphors tend to subvert what people believe the possible models of things are, and make possible the creation of new kinds of models of things. With the metaphor the body is a machine, machine models of the body became a possibility, replacing, for better or worse, the humoral homeostatic models of the previous age (Bynum and Porter, 1997, chapter 14). Likewise, the metaphor that insanity is a brain disease, or of mental illness, replace earlier conceptualizations, allowing a new kind of model to flourish.

An example of the historical contingency of models is to be found in the psychiatric field, in the genetic model of mental illness. Genetics begins to be associated with mental illness at a particular historical point. Scull (1989, chapter 9) reports that this happened in the second half of the nineteenth century, and was consonant with the diminishment of hopes of curing or even treating mental illness: 'As explanations of mental illness were ever more frequently couched in terms of structural brain disease, defective heredity, and Morelian degeneration, so there emerged an entrenched expectation that most cases of mental illness would prove incurable.' (p. 245; see also Dowbiggin, 1985).

Moreover, as genetics has advanced, so has the nature of genetic models upon which the genetic aspect of schizophrenia has been based. Claridge's hypertension model is a case in point. He thinks that the genetic role will be dispositional. Certainly it has become increasingly appreciated how complex the factors that go into disease may be, including genetic factors. But earlier models of the genetics of schizophrenia may have been rather different (cf. Marshall, 1992, p. 89; Boyle, 1990, p. 118).

In short, models will not stand still because science is always developing and recategorizing things.[1] But the metaphor that madness or lunacy is an illness remains the basis of such specific claims, however they may change in detail through history.

The medical model

I think I need to take one more possible objection to these arguments into account. It is that I have substituted talk of a metaphor for what is most often, and according to the objection, rightly, talk of a model. The objection states that the notion of mental illness is not, contrary to what I seem to have been suggesting, to be thought of as a metaphor. Rather, it is the product of a model, to wit, the medical model of insanity. This is a much larger-scale model than those I have considered, such as those of schizophrenia or manic-depressive illness. None the less, the objection holds it has the same characteristics as those smaller-scale models. Sometimes, a distinction appears to be drawn between the phrase mental illness used literally and referring to something modelled upon the medical, and the phrase mental illness used metaphorically and referring to something modelled on non-medical lines. This is a distinction in which Svensson (1990, pp. 72ff) and Radden (1985, see below) are interested. Svensson holds that mental illness needs to be modelled on something other than illness, and so holds that the metaphorical usage (as he understands it) of mental illness is the correct one (see Chapter 4). If mental illness were really an illness, he implies, then it would rightly be modelled on physical illness or disease, and we would not have a metaphor. This is quite the opposite of what I am arguing. The question arises as to whether calling mental illness a metaphor is a mistake, in the light of the fact that I take this to imply the notion that such things as schizophrenia are literally illnesses.

I think not: and my reason is illustrated when we look more carefully at accounts of the so-called medical model of mental illness. Jennifer Radden, who, like Svensson, has objections to the medical model (or as she calls it the 'disease model') of mental illness, says: 'This model depends on perceived analogies between madness and certain aspects of clinical medicine, such as its view of the disease process, its conception of aetiology, its characteristic practices and procedures and the social attitudes and roles it invites.' (Radden, 1985, p. 14). The model is, she goes on to point out, only as good as the central underlying analogy: 'that between the psychological states and behaviour comprising what can be observed of madness—its manifestations, as I shall call them—and the symptoms of a physical ailment' (p. 15). This granted, she observes, much else follows: 'Madness has physical causes analogous to the causes of physical diseases. It is appropriately treated in a medical setting. Its sufferers are rightly seen as victims of their condition and as blameless for having it. The terminology of "therapy", "cure", "prognosis", etc., and a system of medical nosology, rightly apply.' (*Ibid.*). (This formulation of the medical model Radden bases in part on the work of Veatch (1982).)

Radden's position, that 'madness is a disease' represents a model contrasts with mine, that it is a metaphor. Radden presumably thinks in terms of models because she thinks in terms of analogies. We can rightly model madness upon disease, she argues, provided that the manifestations of madness are analogous to the symptoms of physical disease. I have argued that the analogies are themselves the product of the metaphor that madness is a disease rather than the other way around.

The difficulty with Radden's position from my point of view is with the talk of an analogy between the immediately observable 'psychological states and behaviour' we find in madness and the immediately observable 'symptoms' of a physical disease, such as fever, pain, tiredness, and so on. These can be analogized in two senses, but on inspection neither is of any use to Radden. (1) They might be analogized in the sense of having things in common between them. In this case, it is far from clear what would follow. Things can be like one another without being of the same kind, as the weak view of the mistake in likeness argument insists. It is difficult to see how the consequences Radden refers to would have to follow from an analogy of this kind.

Alternatively, (2) we might say that the immediately observable behaviours of the mad are analogous to the symptoms of illness in virtue of their relation to other aspects of madness, namely those not immediately observable. She cites Bates (1977, p. 10) '[The disease model rests upon] . . . a belief that mental illness is a disease process, with an organic or biochemical underlying cause, with certain symptoms, and specific treatments and prognoses' (p. 14). But this will not do for Radden either, as this presumes the right relation between the observable behaviours and the other aspects of madness. In short it presumes they have the same relation as symptoms have with the physical causes of physical disease. But then the existence of the analogy depends upon the application of the model. And this leaves unanswered what makes possible the application of the model.

It is possible that Radden and I disagree only in our choice of words. And I would say that the relation between models and metaphors is often fluid.[2] What is clear is that, in my terms, her choice of the word model is a mistake. The sort of consequences she believes follow from the analogy between the manifestations of madness and the symptoms of physical disease are much better explained by seeing what she calls the disease model of mental illness as a metaphor.

Metaphors and the theory dependence of observation

We may seem now to be in philosophically well-explored territory. We seem to be saying that observation is not independent of our thoughts, ideas, and attitudes. The models we think appropriate to some situation are based upon our observation of the features of things and that in turn is based upon the kind of thing we think the things in question are. The familiar idea that seems to capture this is that observation is theory dependent or laden.

This idea is almost a truism of the philosophy of science in the later twentieth century. Karl Popper argues that 'our ordinary language is full of theories; that observation is always *observation in the light of theories*' (Popper, 1972, p. 59fn; Popper's italics). That is to say even our day-to-day observations and reactions, and not only our specialized scientific observations, are theory dependent. We see things in the way we see them, expect things to happen in certain ways in the future and so on, because we think of them and understand them in terms of, or under the aspect of, our theories. We see the pram in danger of falling over the cliff edge because we have a theory about heavy wheeled objects rolling down slopes and falling when unsupported. If we did not have such theories we would not see the pram as being in danger of falling.

My thesis is I think consistent with the idea that something other than observation lies behind, or perhaps better *within* observation. However, I have not used the word theory, and this has been a deliberate choice. When arguing that alcoholism, ADHD, and schizophrenia may appear to be illnesses to those who think of the evidence of genetic correlations in the right way I did not say that it would seem that way to those who had a theory that they were illnesses. Again, I took up Szasz's point that we can be interested in the phenomena of so-called mental illnesses in different ways. However, I did not say that we can have different theories about such phenomena. I have argued that if we think of alcoholism as an illness then the evidence of genetic causality may seem clear, or at least worthy of further research and specification. If, on the other hand, we do not think of alcoholism as an illness, the so-called evidence of genetic causality may evaporate in questions about temptation and moral fibre. But once again I did not say that if we had a theory that alcoholism was caused genetically then it would be.

This is because I want to distinguish a change of categorization by a metaphor from a theory. I do not mean to make this a hard and fast distinction, stipulating that this is how we must use the words in future or that this is their true meaning. I am merely using the two different words to denote a distinction. There is a meaning of the word theory that like the words hypothesis and model implies that it can be tested. Some authors use metaphor in effect interchangeably with these terms (cf. MacCormac, 1976, p. 36). And the reverse seems true too: a distinct idea, for which the word theory may also sometimes be used, and for some examples of which I am using the term metaphor, is of a view of things that cannot be tested. It cannot be tested because it lies deep enough in the way we think of and experience things to be beyond any refutation, though it might be rejected or abandoned.

I can illustrate the idea of a theory that lies so deep or is so entrenched in us that it appears to be part of our perception itself from my own experience.

When you first point a sufficiently powerful telescope at Jupiter on a clear night you will see a straight line of small bright objects all relatively near to the planet. You will (if you are anything like me) be astounded to realize you have seen some of the moons of Jupiter for the first time. Seeing them there in a straight line and so proximate to the planet leaves one in absolutely no doubt that it is Jupiter's moons that one has seen. One would want to describe what one had seen in precisely these terms, and one would find it difficult to find any other terms that would, in all seriousness and honesty, describe what one had seen. Yet when people first looked at Jupiter with telescopes it is unlikely that they would have seen anything of that description. The idea that planets had moons was unheard of, certainly not established. They would probably have reacted in a completely different way. For example, the apparent proximity of the moons of Jupiter to the planet which struck me in seeing them might have been absent to someone looking at them in the sixteenth century. Something of what we think we see goes into what we see.

But it does not go into that seeing as an interpretation; or even as a testable theory under which we see. Rather it appears to be part of the seeing, part of the perception. For the kind of experience I have just reported, as for the experience of seeing the pram rolling down the hill, the notion of a theory seems to me potentially unhelpful. I take theory to refer to ideas that have a structure, an intellectual coherence and consistency, and an explanatory and perhaps predictive function. If observation is theory dependent in this sense of theory then that makes the human contribution to what we see rather formal and conscious. There is introduced a gap between the seeing and the interpretation or theorizing of the seeing that I wish to suggest is not necessarily there in much of our seeing, even though we contribute to what we see.

It is into this gap that the notion of testing a theory fits. We can ask whether or not the theory explains or meets with our perceptions. However, a theory, such as the theory of gravity, may become so deeply embedded in our understanding and perception of the world that it simply becomes part of our seeing. Twentieth century people do not see stones falling because they are in direct contact with other things such as the air, as would an Aristotelian physicist (cf. MacCormac, 1976, pp. 122–3). Rather we have accepted the idea of action at a distance. The theory of gravity was once perhaps a conscious effort to rethink the notion of physical movement. But it is not any longer.

This is how I imagine the notion that the body is a machine now strikes anatomists and physiologists; and more directly to our point it is how psychiatrists, and the general public, perceive mental illness. It is as if mental illness is something we are given by the world; something independent of us that actually imposes itself upon us. For me this is also the source of the apparent naturalness or inevitability of an idea that the social constructionist is countering. This is why Szasz's idea that mental illness is a metaphor is so radical, and so counter-intuitive, at least until one has given it due consideration. What we tend to think of as imposed upon us by the world turns out to be imposed on the world by us. But when we do give Szasz's ideas due consideration, we find that the idea that we impose mental illness on the world is not at all implausible. However, we also find that this does not necessarily lead us to sceptical and indeed revisionist conclusions.

Someone may say that the kind of notion that cannot be refuted but only rejected or abandoned is the kind usually called metaphysical. As a metaphor such as madness is illness appears to be beyond test, it is metaphysical. This would be said because one (typically hostile) characterization of metaphysical claims is that they are beyond validation, confirmation, or even falsification. Tests do not touch them. Indeed, it is sometimes said that metaphysical statements are meaningless for precisely the reason that they cannot be tested. That is not an issue I'd like to comment on. Rather I do not think metaphors such as the body is a machine or insanity is purely a disease of the brain are metaphysical in the sense just explained. They are not meaningless. They mean just exactly what they say, even though what they say may seem wrong in the light of our existing categories. But they are beyond refutation because readjusting our categories is not a hypothesis or theory or model of how things are. It is a way of categorizing things. We experience it first in our imagination. Then we may begin to experience the world in that way.

It is, however, this way of thinking that leads to the charge that my account of psychiatry is irrational or non-rational. The charge is that I have based this science upon what can be experienced in the imagination; but this is an unreasonable basis for a science.

8.5 Scientific rationality

I propose simply to accept this charge.

A scientist does not necessarily have to give reasons for everything she does or justify every belief that she holds. Perhaps she would be unable to do so. The idea that the body can be described mechanically may be so deeply embedded within a scientist's thought that it is never questioned, let alone justified. The editors of *Gray's* do refer us to Descartes, but they do not run through his arguments. If they were fully cognisant of their nature we might find that they in fact rejected them. None the less, given they accept Descartes' description of the human body they proceed perfectly rationally. Psychiatrists perhaps rarely take seriously the idea that mental illness does not exist, or question the basic diagnostic categories of mental illness. That is not to say that such beliefs cannot be questioned; perhaps any belief can be questioned in some context. Rather it is to say that scientists often proceed without raising such questions and perhaps without having the ability to respond to them if raised. Their allegiance to the way they believe the world to be does not entail their raising questions about every aspect of their beliefs. Some things they take on trust.

Notwithstanding, even where basic beliefs have been questioned, and indeed overturned, the scientific practices that were based upon them do not seem to be any the less rational or reasonable for that. Newtonian physics seems to have proceeded quite rationally for several generations after Newton. However, when its basic assumptions, such as the absoluteness of time and space, came to be questioned in the nineteenth century, they were found wanting. Nevertheless a scientist may proceed, discovering and solving problems and developing subtheories, though upon the basis of ideas that are, in the final analysis, capable of mutation or outright rejection. Kuhn refers to normal science, which is the continuation of scientific exploration within a particular paradigm. When paradigms change, what is normal changes too (Kuhn, 1970).

In the idea of proceeding, or carrying on a scientific enterprise or practice, however, there does seem to be a difference between scientist and poet. A poet who uses the metaphor 'green thought' (Marvell, 1972, p. 101) need not believe that thoughts really are coloured, nor act upon that. Indeed, it may not be clear what 'acting on' would be in the case of thoughts being coloured. Medical scientists, on the other hand, do tend to believe that the body is a machine, and do act upon that. They write textbooks describing the body in the relevant terms, as we have seen; they teach others to describe the body in this way too; they conduct surgery and treatment on that basis; and so forth. That is to say these metaphors enter the poet's life and the scientist's life in very different ways. That has been the point of the discussion of models in the foregoing.

This is true too of the metaphor of mental illness and the psychiatrist. How exactly psychiatrists carry on once they have categorized lunacy as mental illness depends on how exactly they happen to develop their models, hypotheses, and theories. The early turn to the genetic model went hand in hand with the belief of the time that madness was an incurable condition. The recent turn, as in Claridge's arguments, to the genetic model may go hand in hand with a renewed optimism that what is genetic can be understood and perhaps in some sense avoided or even cured. This is a belief that may have been nurtured by the success of the Human Genome Project in mapping the human genome, which was itself based upon the development of gene mapping technology. However, medical science can develop in unpredictable and unexpected ways. Genetics may be flavour of this month; it does not follow that genetic models will always be in favour.

What cannot be ruled out is that some other and completely different basic metaphor will in the future be applied to those whom we currently say have schizophrenia, manic-depression, and other diagnoses offered by psychiatry. The notion of mental illness may well have become deeply embedded in our view of the world. Like gravity it may appear to be something we simply see. It does not follow that it is immune to changes in our ways of thinking. However deeply ingrained, it represents a way of thinking itself.

Endnotes

1 Two potentially important developments for medicine are systems theory and chaos theory. For the relevance of systems theory to medicine see Querido and Gijn (1994). Systems theory holds that the whole is greater than the sum of its parts (*ibid.*, p. 70). As a result it tends to be opposed to the idea that disease or illness could be explained wholly in terms of the 'break down' of smaller units (e.g. cells) and tries instead to account for things at higher levels, for instance at the level of the sick organism as a whole, and seen in context. A development in the mathematics of chaos (the popular name for non-linear dynamics) is generating models for events that have always seemed beyond the reach of science to predict. Chaos theory arose out of studies of weather systems. But one element of the mathematics of chaos, the mathematics of fractals, has already made an impact on thinking in anatomy and physiology (cf. Goldberger and West, 1987; Velanovich, 1994). And Goldberger has identified what he calls the stereotypical behaviours of obsessive compulsives as a subject for reflection (Goldberger, 1997, p. 543). Goldberger's idea is that there is predictability about the behaviour of an obsessive compulsive person that is lacking in a normal person. But while this is a brand new model for the psychiatrist to consider, it is no less dependent upon the idea of mental illness. It might be that fractals offer a new metaphor for the understanding of the body. One of the oddities about fractal patterns created from mathematical models is that they never get simpler. Rather, within the original complex patterns can be identified areas in which the patterns originally found are exactly reproduced in miniature. And so on *ad infinitum*. And this could be used as a metaphor, replacing the idea that models should explain complex patterns in simpler terms. Foss, (1994, p. 308) also refers to new sciences of the brain. In these, he claims, 'The notion of downward causation is scientifically legitimated and with it the proposition that the disease equation can be solved by acknowledging the interaction of holistic downward causal, i.e. memetic, influences alongside reductionistic upward causal, i.e. genetic, influences.' He mentions the work of Skarda and Freeman (1987), Freeman (1991), and Skarda and Freeman (1990).

2 Lakoff and Johnson speak of 'metaphorical models' (1980, p. 28). Speaking of disease, ten Have uses the terms 'infection model' and 'infection paradigm' interchangeably (ten Have, 1990, p. 17). The dominance and centrality that this idea attained (according to ten Have) suggests the possibility that all attempts to explain specific diseases would need to be judged against it, rather than it being judged against them, which is a strong parallel with my notion of metaphor.

9 Conclusions

At the start of this book, I said I would seek to answer some radical questions. These included Thomas Szasz's question 'Does mental illness exist?' and a number of other questions of a more specific nature such as 'Is there any such thing as schizophrenia' and 'Does ADHD exist'. Thomas Szasz answers his own question 'no'; and writers such as Mary Boyle and Breggin answer no to the more specific questions. This of course makes the radical questions more interesting: if people are willing to give a radical—i.e. negative—answer to them, it seems they are worth careful thought.

Such radical questions invite further questions: In what way do such things as mental illness exist if indeed they do exist? As we have seen, particularly in the last part of the book, but throughout really, there are different ways in which such things may be said to exist. They way I have said they exist—as imaginative categorizations—means in effect that they exist as ideas. These ideas take a medical form, I have argued. That is to say, they involve relations between such things as genes, cells, parts of brains, and so on, and they broadly seek causal explanations of things. The categorization of something—say ADHD behaviours, or what might have been called madness at one time—as an illness involves the construction of concepts and theories in these terms. I used the notion of an internal relation to indicate that a particular set of descriptive resources (such as the concepts and theories of medicine) have been applied to the understanding and exploration of various patterns of behaviour and thought, such as alcohol abuse, or inattentiveness and impulsivity in class or at work, or claims to hear voices or to be some famous historical personage. So, for example, the kinds of descriptions that arise out of categorizing such behavioural patterns as illnesses, may be functional and causal.

I have suggested that it is in the light of such descriptions that doctors and medical scientists and others associated with their enterprise investigate the phenomena, that is to say, the alcohol abuse or whatever. It is also, I have argued, in the light of the idea that these are illnesses that the further phenomena they may uncover are understood. Once something like, say ADHD, is characterized as an illness, the investigations of researchers into its nature will be directed along the sorts of lines that other illness investigations are being conducted. With the current development of methods in human genetics, and the growth of brain scanning technologies, researchers into the nature of ADHD tend to seek these routes to the further understanding of the condition. They interpret what they find in genetic studies and in brain scans in the light of the way they have categorized the object of their study. Evidence from brain scans is deployed to suggest a causal account, for example.

The research into particular subject areas will naturally develop its own ideas and its own evidence in the light of these. That is to say, given the initial categorization, there is no predetermined path along which research into any specific subject must go. Within any specific research field—whether into schizophrenia, ADHD, alcoholism, mania, or whatever—novel ideas may develop. To categorize something as an illness is to determine only at a very general level what understanding of that thing will be pursued. Medicine is itself subject to great internal changes periodically.

It may well be that the way I have construed what a 'yes' answer to the radical questions would be like will appear unhelpful. In effect, my sketch of a positive answer to questions such as 'does mental illness exist' or 'does ADHD exist', is to say that they do when they are thought of as existing. I have said that this means that they exist as human constructs. I have argued that this does not make them social constructs, because I take it that a social construct is made out of social materials. But, all the same, I have not argued that such things as ADHD or schizophrenia exist in some way independently of human construction. The foundation of the existence I have attributed to mental illnesses is not the fabric of nature, but is instead a human woven fabric. I have argued that the materials out of which the weaving has been done are ideas about natural materials. But I have also argued that the meaning of discoveries in terms of those natural materials—discoveries about genes, or psychological or brain processes—is to be found only in the light of the belief that they are illnesses.

If this is the foundation I am offering to psychiatry, one might forgive a psychiatrist for saying that it is little better than the sceptic's rejection of psychiatry. I may seem to have bought into so much of the sceptic's agenda that I can no longer offer psychiatry a basis that any legitimate science could admit to having. As the sceptic's agenda seems to be to show that psychiatry is no science, by showing that it has not got any object to study, but has in fact invented or imagined it, my argument that imagination or invention is the basis of mental illness looks very much like the sceptic's statement with an unconvincing spin put on it.

It may not help, either, if I seek to defend myself from someone who is concerned in this way about my arguments, by saying that I have spoken of the way in which an imaginative idea can become entrenched in our ways of thinking about and perceptions of things around us to such an extent that it appears more or less natural to think of and indeed simply to respond or react to things in that way. The problem with this claim may be that it looks as if it exposes psychiatry to the social constructionist critique. This critique, according to Hacking, makes sense only where something takes on the appearance of being an entirely natural part of the world or of the mind. The social constructionist starts from this point, and aims to show that this naturalness is merely an appearance.

The psychiatrist may well then want something more from someone who appears to be offering a defence of psychiatry than this. However, it does not appear to me to be possible to offer anything more. I shall try to say why. Loughlin (2003) says something apposite and important here. He says that the area in which psychiatry finds itself is inherently a tricky one. It is located at a place where so many different ideas, interests, understandings, and explanations cross one another's paths. This is inevitable given that psychiatry is at the place where brains, behaviours, values, laws, beliefs, society, psychology, and history seem to come together to make humans what they are and what they believe themselves to be. And it is here that all manner of sciences, social sciences, and humanities disciplines may focus their lenses in the study of the human being. These various aspects of humans, as we understand them, and these various means of study of humans that seek to expand and encourage our understandings, are not all, so far, entirely compatible.

So, there is, as things stand, an inherent controversy around how best to understand human behaviour. The clash is well illustrated in Accardo and Blondis's (2000) summary of the history of ADHD. They argue (p. 7) that: 'Although certain psychiatric categories do reflect an inappropriate medicalization of behavior . . . , the misapplication of sociological methods to ADHD can only be accomplished by ignoring a broad base of both clinical and basic research.'

The claim here seems to be that ADHD, at least, does not represent medicalization, and that to claim it does is to misapply a sociological approach to it. The presumption is that there is some way of deciding which is the right method of understanding to apply to something such as ADHD. In the terms sometimes used, we might say their presumption is that there is some way of deciding what sort of interest we should take in such things as madness or particular behaviour patterns. However, it seems to me—and perhaps to Loughlin (2003) too—that this is to fail to come to terms with the nature of the problem of giving an account of human behaviour.

One advantage of the account of mental illness that I have attempted to give, I believe, is that it recognizes these controversies. It is able to give an account of them, and, moreover, this is not a sceptical account. That is to say, it does not favour scepticism about any particular approach. My approach applies as much to the social constructionist as to the medical account. On my approach, all the various accounts of human behaviour—psychological, philosophical, sociological, medical, psychiatric, and so on—work within their own disciplines, their own structures of understanding, their own descriptive resources. And, so far as this goes, none of them is privileged.

This may itself be a basis of a complaint against my approach. Accounts such as the mental illness or ADHD accounts, and the social constructionist account of ADHD for that matter, may hold that they are privileged or that they have a hold of some evidence or reason for granting them a privileged position. Accardo and Blondis cite the research base of their own discipline and in doing so make a claim to the truth of the matter about ADHD and, in the same breath, a claim to knowing the way to get to the truth. They argue that the sociological account can work only by ignoring the clinical and basic research base within the ADHD approach. On the other hand, a social constructionist approach may suggest that ADHD has an extratheoretical function that is not being admitted by those who (naively, perhaps) keep within the theoretical (medical) approach.

However, in making these arguments, the proponents of the various positions, are reflecting, or so I would argue, the implicit assumptions and ideas of their own viewpoint. For example, in suggesting that the sociological account must have ignored the clinical and basic research base by now established for ADHD, Accardo and Blondis are implying that taking it into account would force the sociologist into changing his or her account and perhaps approach. But about this they are wrong. A sociological approach such as that of the social constructionist can accommodate the supposed basic and clinical research into ADHD, as I showed in Chapter 7.

My approach can do too, but without being sceptical about it. The sceptic about mental illness or ADHD seizes upon the idea that the traditional medical account tries to set itself up as the arbiter of truth and rationality. For the sceptic, because this is part and parcel of the medical view of the world, it is suspect. But for me, this is not a reason for scepticism. It is important, I would argue, to suggest that there is a sense in which the medical view in which mental illness and specific diagnoses appear sets out its own criteria for success, and applies its own interpretations to what it sees and finds around it, in the light of its own presuppositions about explanation and understanding. But recognizing this, we have not produced justification for denying the legitimacy of the approach.

Nor does my argument support the idea that science proceeds altogether without reference to what it may discover. A number of the things I have said might seem to support this claim. For example, I have suggested that psychiatry or medical science has a meaning ready for the things it finds. I have also suggested that failure to find the kinds of evidence they may seek to support their ideas—for example, the claim that insanity is a disease of the brain or whatever—has not undermined psychiatrists' belief in those ideas. And I have argued that in any case, the evidence is not actually the basis of psychiatrists' beliefs. But notwithstanding, the ideas that psychiatrists have are framed in such a way that they can be put as questions to the world. And, though they may take predetermined forms, their interpretations are none the less interpretations *of* the things they find. So, it may be that psychiatrists look to genetic information, or brain scans showing physiological brain abnormalities, or other means to find anatomical changes, and that we know in advance that these will be used to provide causal accounts of mental illness or of specific mental illnesses. None the less, the medical scientist cannot invent the genetic, physiological, or anatomical evidence. And it is to these sorts of things that medical scientific constructs lead the scientist.

Loughlin complains that my strong objection to the likeness argument implies that we cannot escape seeing things within our own sets of concepts. My position, at least at that point in my argument, runs the risk of being a sceptical and irrational one. But I think the way I develop the position might be more to Loughlin's liking. Our concepts are not fixed: we develop new ideas (such as Pasteur's notion of vaccination) and new categorizations for things (such as the body or patterns of behaviour). And the ideas that our new conceptualizations may lead to can be formulated in testable ways.

Moreover, our conceptualizations can be undone. They can be replaced when new categorizations come along to challenge the existing ones. So, we are not stuck with our concepts. Indeed, current disagreements over the existence of mental illness, schizophrenia, ADHD, alcoholism, and other psychiatric diagnoses, may represent this sort of challenge. What this book has suggested is that one way of understanding these disagreements is to see in them the varying answers to radical questions, whether about the existence of particular mental illness or mental illness in general, which the human imagination helps to create.

References

Abrams, M.H. (1953). *The Mirror and the Lamp: romantic theory and the critical tradition*. London: Oxford University Press.

Accardo, P.J. and Blondis, T.A. (2000). The Strauss syndrome, minimal brain dysfunction, and the hyperactive child: a historical introduction to attention deficit hyperactivity disorder. In: Accardo, P.J., Blondis, T.A., Whitman, B.Y., and Stein, M.A. (eds), *Attention Deficits and Hyperactivity in Children and Adults: diagnosis-treatment-management* (2nd edn, revised and expanded). New York: Marcel Dekker, Inc., pp. 1–11.

American Psychiatric Association (1987). *Diagnostic and Statistical Manual of Mental Disorders* (3rd revised edition) Washington DC: American Psychiatric Association.

American Psychiatric Association (1994). *Diagnostic and Statistical Manual of Mental Disorders* (4th edn). Washington DC:American Psychiatric Association.

Anton, R. (2001). Pharmacologic approaches to the management of alcoholism. *Journal of Clinical Psychiatry* **62** (Suppl. 20): 11–17.

Arendt, R. (2004). *The Shape of the Galaxy* available at *http://homepage.mac.com/rarendt/Galaxy/mw.html* accessed 11th June 2005.

Aristotle (1941). *Poetics*. In: McKeown, R. (ed.), *The Basic Works of Aristotle*. New York: Random House.

Armstrong, S., Gleitman, L., and Gleitman, H. (1983). What some concepts might not be. *Cognition* **13**: 263–308.

Ausubel, D.P. (1967). Personality disorder *is* disease. In: Scheff, T.J. (ed.), *Mental Illness and Social Processes*. New York: Harper and Row, pp. 254–66.

Ayer, A.J. (1978). *Language, Truth and Logic*. Harmondsworth: Penguin.

Bambrough, R. (1970). Universals and family resemblances. In: Pitcher, G. (ed.), *Modern Studies in Philosophy: Wittgenstein. The Philosophical Investigations*. London: MacMillan and Co Ltd, pp. 186–204.

Barkley, R.A. (1997). *ADHD and the Nature of Self-Control*. New York: The Guilford Press.

Baruch, A. and Treacher, A. (1978). *Psychiatry Observed*. London: Routledge and Kegan Paul.

Bates, E. (1977). *Models of Madness*. St Lucia, Queensland, University of Queensland Press.

Beardsmore, R.W. (1992). The theory of family resemblances. *Philosophical Investigations* **15**: 131–46.

Becker, H.S. (1963). *Outsiders*. New York: Free Press.

Bellaimey, J.E. (1990). Family resemblances and the problem of the under-determination of extension. *Philosophical Investigations* **13**: 31–43.

Belloc, H. (1970). *H. Belloc Complete Verse*. London: Gerald Duckworth and Company Ltd.

Black, M. (1954–55). Metaphor. *Proceedings of the Aristotelian Society* New Series, Vol. LV, pp. 273–94.

Black, M. (1980). How metaphors work: a reply to Donald Davidson. In: Sacks, S. (ed.), *On Metaphor*. Chicago: University of Chicago Press, pp. 181–92.

Blondis, T.A., Snow, J.H., and Accardo, P.J. (2000). Methods for measuring attention deficits with or without hyperactivity-impulsivity. In: Accardo, P.J., Blondis, T.A., Whitman, B.Y., and Stein, M.A. (eds), *Attention Deficits and Hyperactivity in Children and Adults: diagnosis·treatment·management* (2nd edn, revised and expanded). New York: Marcel Dekker, Inc., pp. 163–186.

Bloor, D. (1976). *Knowledge and Social Imagery*. London: Routledge and Kegan Paul.

Bloor, D. (1982). Durkheim and Mauss revisited: classification and the sociology of knowledge. *Studies in the History and Philosophy of Science* **13**(4): 267–97.

Boorse, C. (1977). Health as a theoretical concept. *Philosophy of Science* **44**: 542–73.

Boorse, C. (1982). What a theory of mental health should be. In: Edwards, R.B. (ed.), *Psychiatry and Ethics Insanity, Rational Autonomy, and Mental Health Care*. Buffalo, NY: Prometheus Books, pp. 29–48.

Boorse, C. (1997). A rebuttal on health. In: Humber, J. and Almeder, R. (eds), *What is Disease?* Totowa: Humana Press, pp. 3–134.

Boyers, R. and Orrill, R. (1972). *Laing and Anti-Psychiatry*. Harmondsworth: Penguin Books Ltd.

Boyle, M. (1990). *Schizophrenia: a scientific delusion?* London: Routledge.

Breggin, P.R. (1998). *Talking Back to Ritalin: what doctors aren't telling you about stimulants for children*. Monroe, ME: Common Courage Press.

Brody, H. (1985). Philosophy of medicine and other humanities: toward a wholistic view *Theoretical Medicine* **6**: 243–55.

Brown, W.M. (1985). A critique of three conceptions of mental illness. *The Journal of Mind and Behavior* **6**(4): 553–76.

Bynum, W.F. and Porter, R. (1997). *Companion Encyclopedia of the History of Medicine*. London: Routledge.

Canguilhem, G. (1991). *The Normal and the Pathological*. New York: Zone Books.

Cassel, E.J. (1991). *The Nature of Suffering and the Goals of Medicine*. Oxford: Oxford University Press.

Castel, F., Castel, R., and Lovell, A. (1979). *The Psychiatric Society*. New York: Columbia University Press.

Castel, R. (1983). Moral treatment: mental therapy and social control in the nineteenth century. In: Cohen, S. and Scull, A. (eds), *Social Control and the State*. Oxford: Blackwell, pp. 248–266.

Chalmers, A. (1982). *What Is This Thing Called Science?* St Lucia, Queensland: University of Queensland Press.

Chalmers, A. (1990). *Science and its Fabrication*. Milton Keynes: Open University Press.

Champlin, T.S. (1989). The causation of mental illness. *Philosophical Investigations* **12**: 14–32.

Champlin, T.S. (1996). To mental illness via a rhyme for the eye. In: O'Hear, A. (ed.), *Verstehen and Humane Understanding*. Cambridge: Cambridge University Press, pp. 165–89.

Charlton, W. (1975). Living and dead metaphors. *British Journal of Aesthetics* **15**: 172–8.

Clare, A. (1993). Foreword. In: Jenner, F.A., Monteiro, A.C.D., Zagalo-Cardoso, J.A., and Cunha-Oliveira, J.A. (eds), *Schizophrenia A Disease or Some Ways of Being Human?* Sheffield: Sheffield Academic Press, pp. 7–8.

Claridge, G. (1992). Can a disease model of schizophrenia survive? In: Bentall, R.P. (ed.), *Reconstructing Schizophrenia*. London: Routledge, pp. 157–83.

Clendening, L. (1960). *Source Book of Medical History*. New York: Dover Publications.

Cohen, M. (nd). What you need to know about AD/HD under the Individuals With Disabilities Education Act. Online at *http://www.chadd.org/WEBPAGE.CFT?CAT_ID=5&SUBCAT_ID=22&SEC_ID=0* Accessed 23rd September 2005.

Collins Pocket English Dictionary (1996). Glasgow: HarperCollins Publishers.

Conrad, P. (1976). *Identifying Hyperactive Children: the medicalization of deviant behavior*. Lexington, MA: D.C. Heath and Company.

Conrad, P. and Potter, D. (2000). From hyperactive children to ADHD adults: observations on the expansion of medical categories *Social Problems* **47**(4): 559–82.

Cook, E.H. Jr. (2000). Molecular genetic studies of attention deficit/hyperactivity disorder. In: Accardo, P.J., Blondis, T.A., Whitman, B.Y., and Stein, M.A. (eds), *Attention Deficits and Hyperactivity in Children and Adults: diagnosis·treatment·management* (2nd edn, revised and expanded). New York: Marcel Dekker, Inc., pp. 13–27.

Cooper, D. (1970). *Psychiatry and Anti-Psychiatry*. Frogmore: Paladin.

Crossley, N. (1998). R.D.Laing and the British anti-psychiatry movement: a socio-historical analysis. *Social Science Medicine* **47**(7): 877–89.

Culver, C.M. and Gert, B. (1982). *Philosophy in Medicine*. New York: Oxford University Press.

Davidson, D. (1984). What metaphors mean. In: Davidson, D. (ed.), *Enquiries into Truth and Intepretation*. Oxford: Clarendon Press, pp. 245–64.

Descartes, R. (1981a). *Meditations on First Philosophy*. In: Haldane, E.S. and Ross, G.R.T. (transl.) *The Philosophical Works of Descartes*, Vol. 1. Cambridge: Cambridge University Press, pp. 131–199.

Descartes, R. (1981b). *The Principles of Philosophy*. In: Haldane, E.S. and Ross, G.R.T. (transl.) *The Philosophical Works of Descartes*, Vol. 1. Cambridge: Cambridge University Press, pp. 201–302.

Deveson, A. (1992). *Tell Me I'm Here*. Harmondsworth: Penguin.

Diamond, C. (1991). Secondary sense. In: Diamond, C. (ed.), *The Realistic Spirit*. Cambridge: MA: The MIT Press, pp. 225–41.

Diller, L.H. (1998). *Running on Ritalin: a physician reflects on children, society, and performance in a pill*. New York: Bantam Books.

Donagan, A. (1978). How much neurosis should we bear? In: Engelhardt, H.T. and Spicker, S.F. (eds), *Mental Health: philosophical perspectives*. Dordrecht: D.Reidel Publishing Company, pp. 41–53.

Douglas, M. (1975). *Implicit Meanings. Essays in Anthropology* (part 3). London: Routledge and Kegan Paul.

Dowbiggin, I. (1985). Degeneration and hereditarianism in French mental medicine 1840–90. In: Bynum, W.F., Porter, R., and Shepherd, M. (eds), *An Anatomy of Madness. Essays on the History of Psychiatry. Vol. 1: People and Ideas*. London: Tavistock Publications, pp. 188–232.

Drury, M.O.C. (1996). *The Danger of Words and Writings on Wittgenstein*. Bristol: Thoemmes Press.

Dubos, R. (1961). *Pasteur and Modern Science*. London: Heinemann Educational Books Ltd.

Durkheim, E. and Mauss, M. (1903). De quelques formes primitives de classification *Anneé Sociologique 1901–2* (translated and introduced by Needham, R. *Primitive Classification*. London: Cohen and West, 1963).

Elliott, C. (2003). *Better Than Well: American medicine meets the American dream*. New York: W.W. Norton & Company.

Empson, W. (1951). Metaphor. In: Empson, W. (ed.), *The Structure of Complex Words*. London: Chatto and Windus, pp. 331–49.

Engelhardt, H.T. (1984). Clinical problems and the concept of disease. In: Nordenfelt, L. and Lindahl, B.I.B. (eds), *Health, Disease, and Causal Explanations in Medicine*. Dordrecht: D. Reidel Publishing Company, pp. 27–41.

Erikson, K (1966). *Wayward Puritans*. New York: Wiley.

Fleck, L. (1986). To look, to see, to know. In: Cohen, R.S. and Schelle, T. (eds), *Cognition and Fact—Materials on Ludwig Fleck*. Dordrecht: D.Reidel Publishing Company, pp. 129–51.

Flew, A. (1973). *Crime or Disease?* New York: Barnes and Noble.

Foot, P. (ed.) (1978). Moral beliefs. In: *Virtues and Vices*. Oxford: Basil Blackwell, pp. 110–31.

Forman, M. (Director) (1975). *One Flew Over the Cuckoo's Nest*. Los Angeles, United Artists/Fantasy Films.

Foss, L. (1994). Putting the mind back into the body a successor scientific medical model. *Theoretical Medicine* **15**(3): 291–313.

Foucault, M. (1965). *Madness and Civilisation*. London: Tavistock.

Frame, J. (1990). *The Complete Autobiography*. London: The Women's Press.

Freeman, W.J. (1991). The physiology of perception. *Scientific American* **264**(2): 78–85.

Freidson, E. (1970). *Profession of Medicine: a study in the applied sociology of knowledge*. New York: Dodd, Mead.

Frith, C. (1992). *The Cognitive Neuropsychology of Schizophrenia*. Hove: Lawrence Erlbaum Associates, Publishers.

Fukuyama, F. (2002). *Our Posthuman Future: consequences of the biotechnology revolution*. New York: Farrar, Straus and Giroux.

Fulford, K.W.M. (1989). *Moral Theory and Medical Practice*. Cambridge: Cambridge University Press.

Fulford, K.W.M. (2001). 'What is (mental) disease?': an open letter to Christopher Boorse. *Journal of Medical Ethics* **27**: 80–5.

Gipps, R. (2003). Illnesses and likenesses. *Philosophy, Psychiatry, & Psychology* **10**: 255–9.

Goffman, E. (1961). *Asylums*. Harmondsworth: Penguin.

Goldberger, A.L. (1997). Fractal variability versus pathologic periodicity: complexity loss and stereotypy in disease. *Perspectives in Biology and Medicine* **40**(4): 543–61.

Goldberger, A.L. and West, B.J. (1987). Fractals in physiology and medicine. *Yale Journal of Biology and Medicine* **60**: 421–35.

Hacking, I. (1983). *Representing and Intervening Introductory Topics in the Philosophy of Natural Science*. Cambridge: Cambridge University Press.

Hacking, I. (1999). *The Social Construction of What?* Cambridge MA: Harvard University Press.

Hanfling, O. (1981). Introduction. In: Hanfling, O. (ed.), *Essential Readings in Logical Positivism*. Oxford: Basil Blackwell, pp. 1–25.

Harré, R. (1985). *The Philosophies of Science*. Oxford: Oxford University Press.

Harvey, W. (1928). Anatomical studies on the motion of the heart and blood (transl. Leake, C.). Springfield, IL: Charles Thomas (Originally *Exercitatio Anatomica de Motu Cordis et Sanguinis in Animalibus* 1628).

Healy, D. (1990). *The Suspended Revolution: psychiatry and psychotherapy re-examined*. London: Faber and Faber.

Hesse, M. (ed.) (1980). The explanatory function of metaphor. In: *Revolutions and Reconstructions in the Philosophy of Science*. Brighton: Harvester, pp. 111–24.
Hobbes, T. (1975). *Leviathan*. Harmondsworth: Penguin Books.
Hoggett, B. (1996). *Mental Health Law* (4th edn). London: Sweet and Maxwell.
Ingleby, D. (ed.) (1981). *Critical Psychiatry*. Harmondsworth: Penguin.
Ingleby, D. (1983). Mental health and social order. In: Cohen, S. and Scull, A. (eds), *Social Control and the State*. Oxford: Blackwell, pp. 141–188.
Jaspers, K. (1997). *General Psychopathology* (transl. J. Hoenig & M.W. Hamilton). Baltimore: The John Hopkins University Press (1st edn *Allgemeine Psychopathologie* Berlin, Springer, 1913).
Jenner, F.A., Monteiro, A.C.D., Zagalo-Cardoso, J.A., and Cunha-Oliveira, J.A. (1993). *Schizophrenia: a disease or some ways of being human?* Sheffield: Sheffield Academic Press.
Jones, R.M. (ed.) (1984). *Mental Health Act Manual* (4th edn). London: Sweet and Maxwell.
Kant, I. (1961). *Critique of Pure Reason* (transl. Kemp Smith, N.). London: Macmillan and Co. Ltd.
Keefe, R. and Harvey, P. (1994). *Understanding Schizophrenia: a guide to the new research on causes and treatment*. New York: The Free Press.
Keil, F.C. (1992). *Concepts, Kinds, and Development*. Cambridge, MA: The MIT Press.
Kendell, R.E. (1975). The concept of disease and its implications for psychiatry. *British Journal of Psychiatry* **127**: 305–15.
Kesey, K. (1973). *One Flew Over the Cuckoo's Nest*. New York: Viking Press.
Kety, S. (1974). From rationalisation to reason. *American Journal of Psychiatry* **131**: 957–63.
Kety, S. (1985). Schizotypal personality disorder: an operational definition of Bleuler's latent schizophrenia. *Schizophrenia Bulletin* **11**: 590–4.
Knorr-Cetina, K.D. (1983). The ethnographic study of scientific work: towards a constructivist interpretation of science. In: Knorr-Cetina, K.D. and Mulkay, M. (eds). *Science Observed: perspective in the social study of science*. London: Sage, pp. 115–40.
Kuhn, T.S. (1970). *The Structure of Scientific Revolutions*. Chicago: The University of Chicago Press.
Kupfer, D.J. (1991). Biological markers of depression. In: Feighner, J.P. and Boyer, W.F. (eds), *The Diagnosis of Depression*. Chichester, John Wiley and Sons, pp. 79–98.
Laing, R.D. (1964). *The Divided Self* (2nd edn). Harmondsworth: Penguin.
Lakoff, G. and Johnson, M. (1980). *Metaphors We Live By*. Chicago: University of Chicago Press.
Lanczik, M. and Beckmann, H. (1991). Historical aspects of affective disorders. In: Feighner, J.P. and Boyer W.F. (eds), *Diagnosis of Depression*. Perspectives in Psychiatry, Vol. 2. Chichester: John Wiley and Sons, pp. 1–16.
Latour, B. (1993). *We Have Never Been Modern* (transl. Porter, C.). Cambridge, MA: Harvard University Press.
Lessing, D. (1971). *Briefing For A Descent Into Hell*. London: Cape.
Lewis, C.S. (1981). *The Pilgrim's Regress*. New York: Bantam.
Lock, T.M. and Bender, D.B. (2000). Single neuron studies of attention. In: Accardo. P.J., Blondis, T.A., Whitman, B.Y., and Stein, M.A. (eds), *Attention Deficits and Hyperactivity in Children and Adults: diagnosis·treatment·management* (2nd edn, revised and expanded). New York: Marcel Dekker, Inc., pp. 29–56.

Loughlin, M. (2003). Contingency, arbitrariness and failure. *Philosophy, Psychiatry, & Psychology* **10**: 261–6.

MacCormac, E.R. (1976). *Metaphor and Myth in Science and Religion*. Durham, NC: Duke University Press.

McKinney, K. (nd). What is a planet? *New Zealand Astronomical Yearbook 2005*, 16–19.

Macklin, R. (1981). Mental health and mental illness: some problems of definition and concept formation. In: Caplan, A., Engelhardt Jr., H., and McCartney, J. (eds), *Concepts of Health and Disease. Interdisciplinary Perspectives*. Reading, MA: Addison-Wesley Publishing Company, pp. 391–418.

Mannheim, K. (1952). The problem of a sociology of knowledge. In: Mannheim, K. (edited and translated Kecskemeti, P.) *Essays on the Sociology of Knowledge*. London: Routledge and Kegan Paul Ltd (originally published in *Archiv für Sozialwissenschaft und Sozialpolitik* Tübingen, **3**(3): 1925).

Margolis, J. (1980). The concept of mental illness: a philosophical examination. In: Brody, B. and Engelhardt Jr, H. (eds), *Mental Illness: law and public policy*. Dordrecht: D. Reidel Publishing Company, pp. 3–23.

Marshall, R. (1992). The genetics of schizophrenia: axiom or hypothesis? In: Bentall, R.P. (ed.), *Reconstructing Schizophrenia*. London: Routledge, pp. 89–117.

Marvell, A. (1972). The garden. In: *The Complete Poems*. Harmondsworth: Penguin, pp. 100–2.

Mercugliano, M. (2000). The neurochemistry of ADHD. In: Accardo, P.J., Blondis, T.A., Whitman, B.Y., and Stein, M.A. (eds), *Attention Deficits and Hyperactivity in Children and Adults: diagnosis·treatment·management* (2nd edn, revised and expanded). New York: Marcel Dekker, Inc., pp. 59–71.

Miller, J. and Szasz, T. (1983). Objections to psychiatry dialogue with Thomas Szasz. In: Miller, J. (ed.), *States of Mind*. London: British Broadcasting Corporation, pp. 270–90.

Miller, P. and Rose, N. (1986). *The Power of Psychiatry*. London: Polity Press.

Murphy, E. (1991). *After the Asylums: community care for people with a mental illness*. London: Faber and Faber.

Pepper, S. (1961). *World Hypotheses A Study in Evidence*. Berkeley: University of California Press.

Phillips, D.Z. (1996). *Introducing Philosophy*. Oxford: Blackwell.

Pickering, N. (1996). Naturally conceived: the idea of the natural in debates about assisted conception. In: Evans, D. (ed.), *Creating the Child*. The Hague: Kluwer Law International, pp. 111–25.

Pickering, N. (1999). Metaphors and models in medicine. *Theoretical Medicine and Bioethics* **20**: 361–75.

Pickering, N. (2003). The likeness argument and the reality of mental illness. *Philosophy, Psychiatry, & Psychology* **10**(3): 243–54.

Pilgrim, D. (1992). Competing histories of madness Some implications for modern psychiatry. In: Bentall, R.P. (ed.), *Reconstructing Schizophrenia*. London: Routledge, pp. 211–33.

Popper, K. (1972). *The Logic of Scientific Discovery* (revised edition). London: Hutchinson and Co. Ltd.

Porter, R. (1988). Introduction. In: Haslam, J. *Illustrations of Madness* (ed. Porter, R.). London: Routledge.

Porter, R. (ed.) (1991). *The Faber Book of Madness*. London: Faber and Faber.

Querido, A. and van Gijn, J. (1994). The wisdom of the body: the usefulness of systems thinking for medicine. In: van Es, L.A. and Mandema, E. (eds), *The Discipline of Medicine. Emerging concepts and their impact upon medical research and medical education*. North-Holland, Amsterdam; Elsevier Science Publishers b.v., pp. 67–78.

Radden, J. (1985). *Madness and Reason*. London: George Allen Unwin.

Ramon, S. (1985). *Psychiatry in Britain*. London: Croom Helm.

Reznek, L. (1991). *The Philosophical Defence of Psychiatry*. London: Routledge.

Richards, I.A. (1936). *The Philosophy of Rhetoric*. New York: Oxford University Press.

Rorty, R. (1980). *Philosophy and the Mirror of Nature*. Oxford: Blackwell.

Rorty, R. (1991). *Objectivity, Relativism, and Truth*. Cambridge: Cambridge University Press.

Rorty, R. (1995). The contingency of language. In: Goodman, R. (ed.), *Pragmatism: a reader*. London: Routledge, pp. 107–23.

Rosch, E. (1977). Human categorization. In: Weil, W. (ed.), *Studies In Cross Cultural Psychology*, Vol. 1. London: Academic Press, pp. 1–49.

Ryan, A. (1970). *Philosophy of the Social Sciences*. London: Macmillan.

Ryan, W. (1971). *Blaming the Victim*. New York: Vintage.

Ryle, G. (1973). *The Concept of Mind*. Harmondsworth: Penguin.

Sarbin, T. (1969). On the scientific status of the mental illness metaphor. In: Plog, S.C. and Edgerton, R.B. (eds), *Changing Perspectives in Mental Illness*. New York: Holt, Rinehart and Winston, pp. 9–31.

Scull, A. (1979). *Museums of Madness*. London: Allen Lane.

Scull, A. (1989). *Social Order/Mental Disorder Anglo-American Psychiatry in Historical Perspective*. London: Routledge.

Sedgwick, P. (1982). *Psychopolitics*. London: Pluto Press.

Shapin, S. and Schaffer, S. (1985). *Leviathan and the Air-Pump: Hobbes, Boyle and the experimental life*. Princeton, NJ: Princeton University Press.

Shelley, P.B. (1947). A defence of poetry. In: Brett-Smith, H.F.B. (ed.), *Peacock's Four Ages of Poetry. Shelley's Defence of Poetry. Browning's Essay on Shelley*. (2nd edn). Oxford: Basil Blackwell, pp. 23–59.

Sieg, K. (2000). Neuroimaging and attention deficit hyperactivity disorder. In: Accardo, P.J., Blondis, T.A., Whitman, B.Y., and Stein, M.A. (eds), *Attention Deficits and Hyperactivity in Children and Adults: diagnosis-treatment-management* (2nd edn, revised and expanded). New York: Marcel Dekker, Inc., pp. 73–117.

Singh, I. (2002). Bad boys, good mothers, and the 'miracle' of Ritalin. *Science in Context* **15**(4): 577–603.

Skarda, C.A. and Freeman, W.J. (1987). How brains make chaos in order to make sense of the world *Behavioral and Brain sciences* **10**: 161–244.

Skarda, C.A. and Freeman, W.J. (1990). Chaos and the new science of the brain. *Concepts in Neuroscience* **1**(2): 275–85.

Smith, D.E. (1978). 'K. is mentally ill' the anatomy of a factual account. *Sociology* **12**: 23–53.

Soskice, J.M. (1989). *Metaphor and Religious Language*. Oxford: Clarendon Press.

Still, G.F. (1902). The Coulstonian Lectures on Some Abnormal Psychical Conditions in Children *The Lancet* (Lecture 1) 12 April, pp. 1008–12; (Lecture 2) 19 April, pp. 1077–82; (Lecture 3) 26 April, pp. 1163–1168.

Svensson, T. (1990). *On the Notion of Mental Illness*. Linköping University: Department of Health and Society.

Szasz, T. (1973). *The Manufacture of Madness*. St Albans, Paladin.
Szasz, T. (1974a). *The Myth of Mental Illness Foundations of a Theory of Personal Conduct* (revised edition). New York: Harper and Brown.
Szasz, T. (1974b). *The Second Sin*. London: Routledge and Kegan Paul.
Szasz, T. (1979). *Schizophrenia*. Oxford: Oxford University Press.
Szasz, T. (1982). The myth of mental illness. In: Edwards, R.B. (ed.), *Psychiatry and Ethics Insanity, Rational Autonomy and Mental Health Care*. Buffalo, NY: Prometheus Books, pp. 19–28.
Szasz, T. (1987). *Insanity: the idea and its consequences*. New York: Wiley.
Szasz, T. (1996). 'Audible thoughts' and 'speech defect' in schizophrenia: a note on reading and translating Bleuler. *British Journal of Psychiatry* **168**: 533–5.
Szasz, T. (2001). Mental illness: psychiatry's phlogiston. *Journal of Medical Ethics* **27**: 297–301.
Szasz, T. (2002). Reply to Brassington. *Journal of Medical Ethics* **28**: 124–5.
ten Have, H.A.M.J. and Henk M.J. (1990). Knowledge and practice in European medicine. In: ten Have, H.A.M.J., Kimsma, G.K. and Spicker, S.F. (eds), *The Growth of Medical Knowledge*. Dordrecht: Kluwer Academic Publishers, pp. 15–40.
Timimi, S. and Taylor, E. (2004). ADHD is best understood as a cultural construct [In Debate]. *British Journal of Psychiatry* **184**: 8–9.
Tirrell, L. (1991). Reductive and nonreductive simile theories of metaphor. *The Journal of Philosophy* **LXXXVIII**(7): 337–58.
Turbayne, C.M. (1970). *The Myth of Metaphor* (revised edition). Columbia: University of South Carolina Press.
Veatch, R.M. (1982). The medical model: its nature and problems. In: Edwards, R. (ed.), *Psychiatry and Ethics Insanity, Rational Autonomy, and Mental Health Care*. New York: Prometheus Books, pp. 88–108.
Velanovich, V. (1994). Reductionism in biology and medicine: theoretical considerations and a practical example. *Theoretical Surgery* **9**: 104–7.
Verwey, G. (1990). Medicine, anthropology, and the human body. In: ten Have, H.A.M.J., Kimsma, G.K., and Spicker, S.F. (eds), *The Growth of Medical Knowledge*. Dordrecht: Kluwer Academic Publishers, pp. 133–62.
Vietnam Veterans of America (2004). VVA's guide on PTSD. Online at *http://www.vva.org/benefits/ptsd.htm*. Accessed 23rd September 2005.
Vogel, F. and Propping, P. (1981). The electroencephalogram (EEG) as a research tool in human behavior genetics. In: Gershon, E.S., Matthysse, S., Breakefield, X.O., and Ciaranello, R.D. (eds). *Genetic Research Strategies for Psychobiology and Psychiatry*. Pacific Grove, CA: The Boxwood Press.
Wakefield, J.C. (1992a). The concept of mental disorder: on the boundary between biological facts and social values. *American Psychologist* **47**(3): 373–88.
Wakefield, J.C. (1992b). Disorder as harmful dysfunction: a conceptual critique of *DSM-III-R*'s definition of mental disorder. *Psychological Review* **99**(2): 232–47.
Whitbeck, C. (1981). A theory of health. In: Caplan, A.L., Engelhardt, H.T., and McCartney, J.J. (eds), *Concepts of Health and Disease. Interdisciplinary Perspectives*. Reading, MA: Addison-Wesley Publishing Company, pp. 611–26.
Williams, P.L., Warwick, R., Dyson, M., and Bannister, L.H. (eds) (1989). *Gray's Anatomy* (37th edn). Edinburgh: Churchill Livingstone.
Wilson, P. (2004). Challenging science: issues for New Zealand science in the 21st century [review]. *Journal of Bioethical Inquiry* **1**: 57–9.

Winch, P. (1990). *The Idea of a Social Science and Its Relation to Philosophy* (2nd edn). London: Routledge.

Wittgenstein, L. (1975). *Philosophical Remarks* (ed. Rhees, R.; transl. Hargreaves, R. and White. R.). Oxford: Basil Blackwell.

Wittgenstein, L. (1992). *Philosophical Investigations* (3rd edn, transl. Anscombe, G.E.M.). Oxford: Basil Blackwell.

Wulff, H.R. (1994). The disease concept and the medical view of man. In: Querido, A., van Es, L.A. and Mandema, E. (eds), *The Discipline of Medicine. Emerging concepts and their impact upon medical research and medical education.* North Holland, Amsterdam: Elsevier Science Publishers bv, pp. 11–19.

Zametkin, A.J., Nordahl, T.E., Gross, M., King, A.C., Semple, W.E., Rumsey, J., Hamburger, S., and Cohen R.M. (1990). Cerebral glucose metabolism in adults with hyperactivity of childhood onset. *New England Journal of Medicine* **323**(20): 1361–6.

Index

July 21 - Aug 7

Socrates

moral treatment 107

insanity was a disease 104

DSM - physical pathology underlies 130

social judgement of deviance 136

meanings to life 154

morality - psychiatry 175

theory dependence of observation 167

Psychiatry is at the place 175